# Retrain The Brain—The Dunn Method

Before we get started, I wanted to share a few things. First of all, this book is not about research or what has been proven or disproven with science. Many things that I was taught in Physical Therapy school in the 90's have since been debunked by science. Things that I learned in the early 2000's have also been debunked and now the evidence has shifted again. I know that PT's that read this book will attack The Dunn Method and that is fine. This is about the success of my clients and what helped them, not what my col-leagues think. Second, I studied all the research in my Manual Therapy Certification with The Maitland Approach (COMT) and didn't get the results that I expected to get. Then I studied Pilates, which opened my mind to the whole body approach. This was the exact opposite of manual therapy that was looking at one specific joint as the problem. With an introduction to the fascial system from John F Barnes and Thomas Myers, it all started to make sense to me. This book combines everything that has worked well for my clients since 2004. It is a simple philosophy that I follow. Release what is locked short and tight. Then strengthen the tissue that is locked long and weak. If we only release or loosen the tight tissue without getting the antagonist muscles stronger, it does not work. If we only strengthen the weak muscles without taking the time to loosen up those opposite tight muscles, that won't work. But if we combine the two, we get much better and lasting results. If you are a person suffering from back pain, this could be the most important book you have ever read. If you are an open minded Physical Therapist, please continue on.

Health Disclaimer:

We make every effort to ensure that we accurately represent the injury advice and prognosis displayed throughout this book. However, examples of injuries and their prognosis are based on typical representations of those injuries that we commonly see in our physical therapy clinic. The information given is not intended to apply to every individual's potential injury. As with any injury, each person's symptoms can vary widely and each person's recovery from injury can also vary depending upon background, family history, past medical history, surgical history, exercise history, posture, motivation to follow through with the advice of the physical therapist and various other physical factors. It is impossible to give a 100% accurate diagnosis and prognosis without a thorough physical examination. The advice given for management of an injury cannot be deemed fully accurate in the absence of an examination from one of our Licensed Physical Therapist at CORE Therapy & Pilates. We are able to offer you this service at a standard charge. Significant injury risk is possible if you do not follow due diligence and seek suitable professional advice about your injury. No guarantees of specific results are expressly made or implied in this book.

# Table of Contents

- BEING MINDFUL OF THE BASICS: LET'S

  BUILD TO DYNAMIC EXERCISE...

  - Ball Squeeze
  - Hip ABD/ER or Clam
  - Alternating March or Tiny Steps
  - Bridging
  - Scapula Setting
  - Foam Roller Lat Pull
  - Foam Roller Horizontal ABD
  - Foam Roller Rotator Cuff
  - Quadruped Co-Contraction
  - Quadruped Leg Lifts
  - Quadruped Arm Lifts
  - Quadruped Alternating Arm and Leg Lifts
  - Sitting Foam Roller Lat Pull
  - Sitting Foam Roller Rows
  - Sitting Lat Pull and Rows
  - Standing Co-Contraction
  - Standing Lat Pull
  - Standing Row

- CHAPTER FOUR

  - APPLYING CORE STRENGTH TO YOUR DAY

    TO DAY LIFE, SPORTS, AND RECREATION

  - Dowel Standing Exercise

# Chapter One

# Release Your Fascia

It was May 1996, my first day of Physical Therapy school and my first class, gross anatomy. After a short lecture, our professor told us to go to the anatomy lab, pick a cadaver and get ready to start our first dissection. We set up in groups of four, lifted our cadaver from the formaldehyde, flipped him over to his stomach, and started our dissection. The first thing our professor said was, "Get rid of the fascia so that we can get to the important anatomy." What he was saying was get rid of the junk so we can see the inner muscles, the nerves, the tendons, the ligaments, the bones, the organs, etc. After the entire semester, I had a five-gallon bucket of fascia that I had removed from my 150-pound cadaver. Over 20 years later, I wonder what it would have been like to study the body without removing the fascia.

What is fascia? Fascia is a three-dimensional spider web that goes throughout the body. The fascia surrounds the muscles, the nerves, the intestines, and the organs. It's between the muscles and the skin. It's everywhere. Fascia has been compared to the packing peanuts we find in our boxes shipped to us from companies like Amazon. The peanuts fill in space in the box to keep everything protected and in the proper place.

Fascia serves a very similar purpose in the body. It separates the layers of muscles to keep them in line doing what they should do. It keeps the muscles in their proper place.

In March of 2018, a new organ called Interstitium was introduced by science. Wikipedia states: The **interstitium** is a contiguous fluid-filled space existing between the skin and the body organs, including muscles and the circulatory system. The fluid in this space is called **interstitial** fluid (or lymph), which is composed of extracellular fluid and its solutes.

The USA Today shared this article on 3/28/18 (https://www.usatoday.com/story/news/health/2018/03/28/study-says-we-have-undiscovered-organ-its-called-interstitium/465173002/)

The NY Times had this to say on 3/31/18 (https://www.nytimes.com/2018/03/31/health/new-organ-interstitium.html?searchResultPosition=1)

# Retrain The Brain—The Dunn Method

**Full Quote from Myofascial Release pioneer John F. Barnes to SmartHer News** (https://smarthernews.com/18-03-29-new-organ/)

*"It is refreshing to see science is finally catching up to what I've been teaching in my Myofascial Release seminars for the last 40 years. The fascial system is one of the most important structures of our body and is significantly tightened from physical or emotional trauma, which produces crushing pressure on pain sensitive structures. It produces symptoms of pain, headaches, fibromyalgia and a myriad of women's pain and health problems. The fascinating fascia is a liquid crystal three-dimensional web. In the space of the web, which is actually not space, but a fluid/viscous substance called the ground substance, the fascia tends to solidify due to trauma, and is the main transport medium of our body. This means that whatever nutrition we ingest, the fluid we drink, the air we breathe, all the biochemistry hormones and information/energy that every one of the trillions of cells needs to thrive must go through the fluidity of the fascia."*

*"I would highly recommend purchasing Dr. Jean-Claude Guimberteau's book, Architecture of Human Living Fascia. He is a French hand surgeon and he represents over 20 years of research on the fascial system. If you go to page 163, I have provided a more detailed explanation of the fascial system and Myofascial Release."*

- John F. Barnes

# Retrain The Brain—The Dunn Method

Here is my blog on it as it hit the news...
(https://therapyandpilates.com/interstitium-science-has-found-a-new-organ-in-2018-we-call-it-fascia-have-been-treating-it-for-15-years/)

The fascial system connects every system in the body, the musculoskeletal system, the nervous system, the cardiovascular system, etc., etc., etc. However, it's the one system that's not tested in modern medicine. Fascia cannot be tested with an MRI, a CT scan, an X-Ray, or with bone density testing. Basically, there is no way to test the fascia in our current medical system. There is no way currently for medical professionals to profit financially from testing the fascia.

Fascia can be tested by a hands-on assessment. By palpating and feeling the fascia and the tissue, you are able to determine where the restrictions are. A postural assessment with a visual inspection of postural imbalances is also important to determine fascial restrictions. Looking at the position of the pelvis, the scapula, the head and the spine one can tell a lot about fascial restrictions.

Many people do not respond to strength training because of fascial restrictions throughout their body. Therefore, we must release these fascial restrictions before strengthening the body. By releasing fascial restrictions, we will create a better and improved posture of the pelvis and spine. This will allow strength training to have a positive and lasting impact.

How do I release my fascia? Hands-on treatment by a skilled therapist is the ideal place to start. Then performing a home program to continue to release the fascia is the next step. Now let's discuss the home exercise program to release your fascia daily. First, you'll need a four-inch inflatable ball. We call it the gold ball here at CORE Therapy and Pilates. Second, you'll need a tennis ball and possibly something firmer like a La Crosse ball.

Get your 4" ball from our Amazon affiliate link at... (https://amzn.to/2Ydl0Fv)

Get your La Cross ball set at... (https://amzn.to/2E1YZUE)

## Psoas

First, we want to release the psoas. This is my favorite. The psoas is a hip flexor that will bring the knee towards the chest in standing. It is deep under the abdominals and the intestines and sits on both sides of the spine. It gets tight and restricted with sitting and we all sit too much today. When the psoas is tight, it pulls the spine into a swayback or an increased lordosis or an arch. To release the psoas, lay on your stomach and place the four-inch gold ball about an inch to the side of your belly button, maybe two inches.

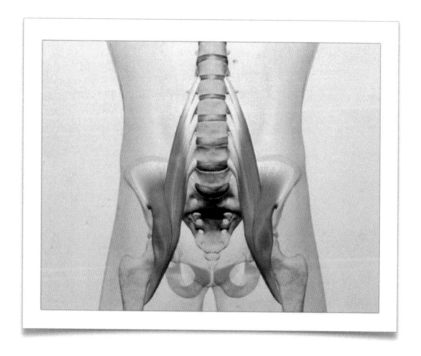

## Retrain The Brain—The Dunn Method

Take a deep breath and your body will rise off the ball. Then exhale and your body will sink deep into the ball, causing pain if you are on the psoas. You may need to move it out half an inch, or up an inch, or down an inch. Once you find that spot that hurts on the exhale, breathe deeply for up to five minutes or when the tension improves and the pain subsides. It may take longer on one side compared to the other as one side is probably tighter and more of a problem.

# Retrain The Brain—The Dunn Method

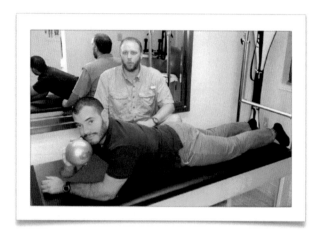

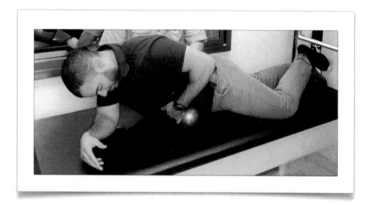

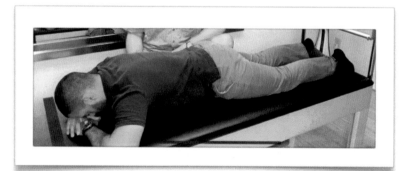

The more you do this release, the faster the pain will subside. After you feel an improvement in the initial discomfort of the psoas you will move on to a series of movements with your legs. If you have the ball on your right side, just to the right of your belly button, you will move your right leg and vice versa. The first leg movement will be bending your knee and moving your heel to your butt. If this is tender or painful where the ball is, continue that movement until is no longer painful. Do not count. Do it until it feels better. You can count to 20 and 20 may be enough. It may not be enough. It may be that 15 is too many. So do it until it feels better. This is the start of awareness. You are paying attention to how your body feels and how it changes.

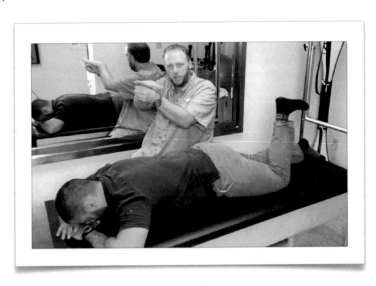

The second motion is to bend the knee to 90 degrees and roll the foot and hip side to side. I call this the windshield wiper. This creates a shifting of the pelvis and causes more pressure on the ball and thus on the psoas as the foot rolls outward. Do this until it feels better just like every self-release movement we will talk about.

# Retrain The Brain—The Dunn Method

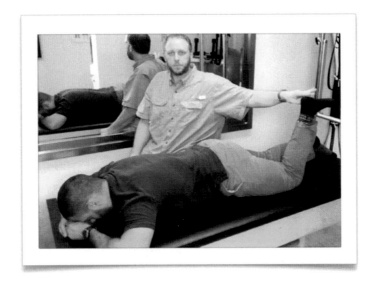

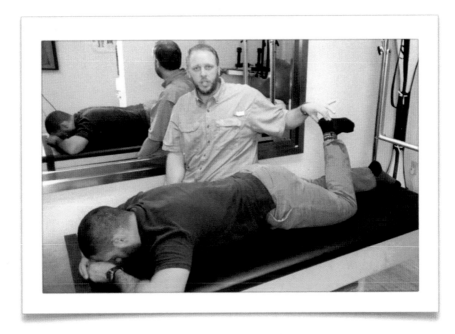

Retrain The Brain—The Dunn Method

The third and final motion in this position is to place your toes into the ground, flexing your foot instead of pointing it. Next, lift your knee off the ground. Do not lift the toes, just the knee. Lower the knee to the ground and repeat. This will drive the ball deeper into the psoas.

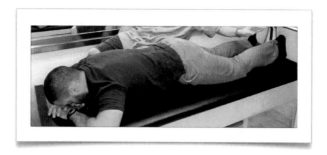

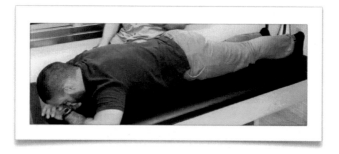

Now repeat this entire sequence on the other side. Remember to keep the ball in line with the belly button.

To access the video to each home exercise, visit the link: https://pilatestothrive.com/backpain/

## Iliacus

Our second muscle to release is the iliacus, also a hip flexor. It attaches to the pelvis, not the spine, and comes down and attaches to the hip bone. To release the iliacus, we will use a tennis ball. If this is too intense, use a piece of pool noodle, cut about three inches long. Lie on your stomach and place the tennis ball just inside your pelvic bone. Do not place the ball on the bone. Repeat the leg movements as you did for the psoas: bending the knee; the windshield wiper; and lifting the knee with the toes into the ground. Do this on both sides. This will likely be painful.

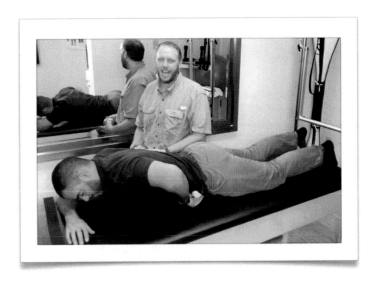

## The Hip Flexor Kickstand

As your hip flexors respond favorably to the release work, it is frequent to feel like the gold ball is no longer providing enough pressure. This is a great sign! Now it is time to do what we call the kickstand. If the ball is under your left hip flexor, psoas or iliacus, take your right leg out to the side while you bend your knee. This will create a shift in your pelvis and increase the tension or pain in the hip flexor. Now do your deep breathing and your leg movements in this kickstand position.

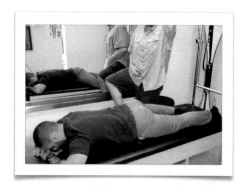

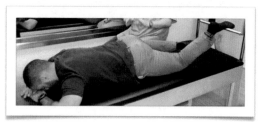

## Diaphragm

The third area to release is the respiratory diaphragm directly under the ribs. This muscle runs side to side and front to back and is shaped like a dome. The diaphragm is responsible for breathing. Most people breathe very shallow and only use the upper third of their lungs. The lower third of the lungs are down at the bottom of the ribs. So how do we release the diaphragm?

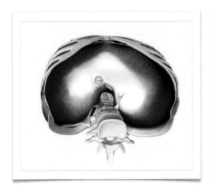 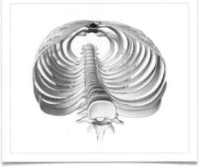

Lay on your stomach. Place the four-inch ball under the rib cage. Start on the left side. The key is to prop up on your elbows and get the ball up and under your ribs. This is a little tricky and is also fairly painful if you place to ball correctly. Take deep breaths for up to five minutes or until this tension relaxes and releases. Do both sides. You can play around with some of the same leg movements from the psoas and iliacus exercises. Move one leg at a time, or move both legs at the same time. This is an important step for the breathing exercises we will work on in later chapters. Proper breathing is very important to strengthening the core.

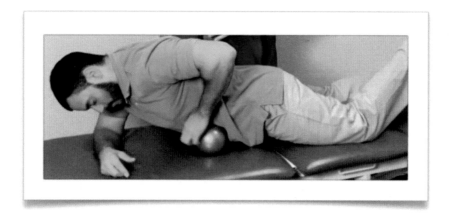

# Retrain The Brain—The Dunn Method

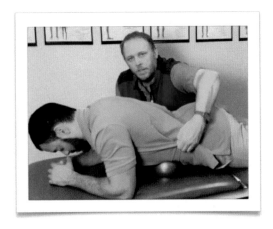

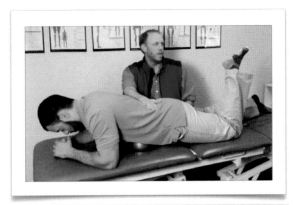

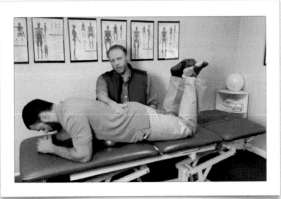

# Retrain The Brain—The Dunn Method

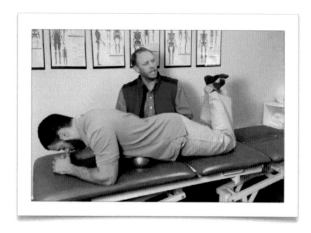

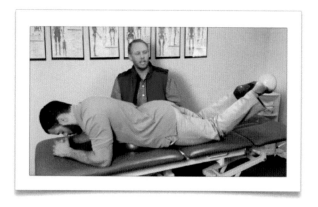

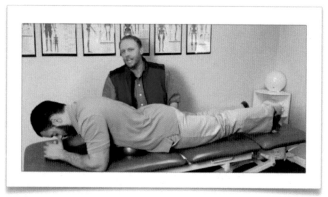

## Pectoralis Minor

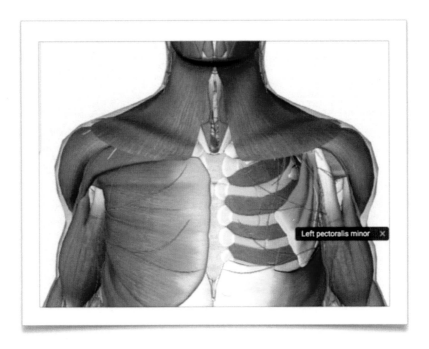

The fourth structure to release for the home program is the pectoralis minor. This is the last structure in the front of the body that ties together the entire anterior tightness resulting from our modern culture of sitting. The pectoralis minor runs from the upper ribs to the shoulder blade. I like to describe it as the bra strap muscle as it basically sits close to where the bra strap runs. It attaches to the shoulder blade and when it gets tight it pulls the shoulder blades forward or rounds the posture into a slouched position. This is not good for the shoulder, the head, the neck, or the lower back. The pectoral minor is often neglected, as well as the diaphragm, when it comes to treating the lower back.

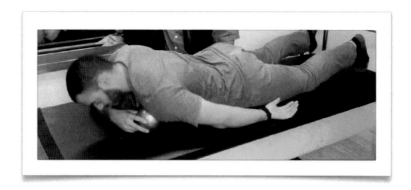

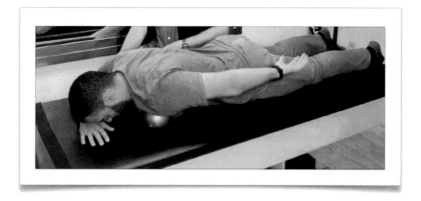

So grab the gold ball and lets try two different options to see what gets the best results. Try lying on your stomach on the floor or standing in a doorframe. Place the ball between the floor or doorframe and your pectoral minor. By using the doorframe you can lean into it. The ball should be under your collarbone, between your armpit and your sternum or the breastbone. If you have the ball on your left pectoral minor, you take your right leg and put it behind your left leg. This would be like stretching your right calf in the runner's stretch position. Push into the floor with your back leg and push into the doorframe pushing into the ball. Next swing that left arm forward and back keeping the elbow straight. This is the same idea as when we were moving the legs and releasing the hip flexors. When that feels better with movement, take your arm and you reach it towards your back pocket. Go up and down, bending your elbow as you reach in and out towards your back pocket. These motions will continue to cause more pressure with the ball at your pectoral minor. Continue these motions until the tension has released. The last motion is reaching overhead.

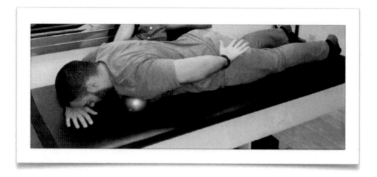

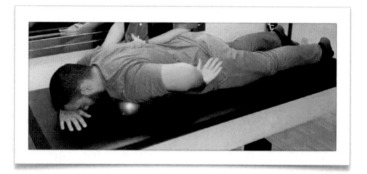

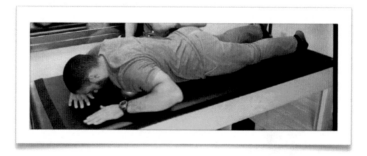

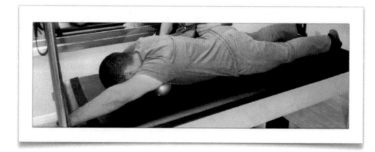

# Retrain The Brain—The Dunn Method

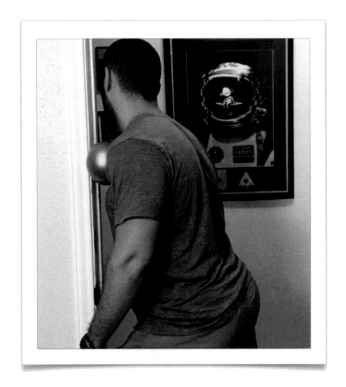

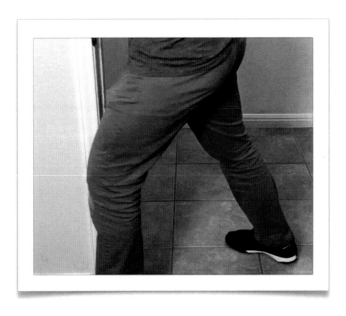

# Retrain The Brain—The Dunn Method

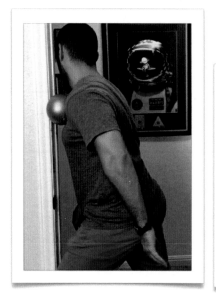

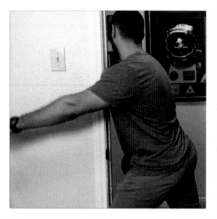

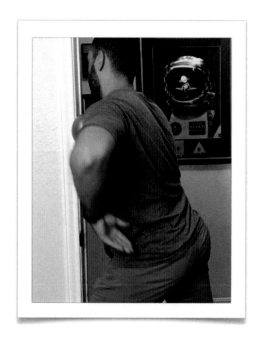

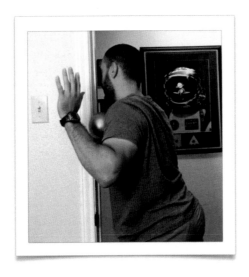

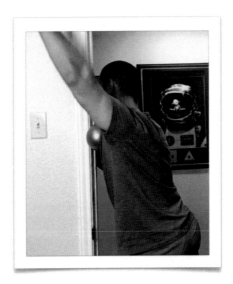

Now I want to discuss two muscles in the back of the body. One is the levator scapulae and the other is the piriformis.

## Levator Scapulae

The levator scapulae attaches from the tip of your shoulder blade close to the neck and runs up to the back of the lower skull. When this muscle gets tight, it elevates the shoulder blade towards the ears. Release the levator by lying on your back on the floor or by leaning into a wall. If on your back, place the tennis ball at the tip of the right shoulder blade. Lift your buttocks and place the foam roller under your pelvis. This will increase the tension on the tight muscle. Now take your right arm and raise it overhead with the elbow straight. This will increase that tension. Continue the movement until the tension releases. The next arm movement is to take the arm to the side of your body like its in a bench press position. Now reach across your body to the left side as you straighten your elbow.

I find it easier to perform this release technique standing at the wall with the ball in a pillowcase or long sock. This will allow you to place the ball over your shoulder without it slipping. Keep your feet 1-2 feet away from the wall.

# Retrain The Brain—The Dunn Method

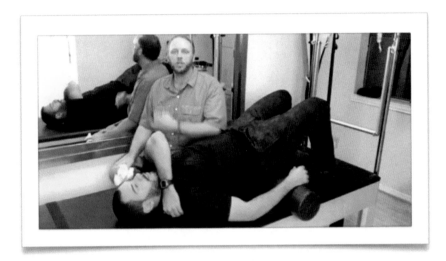

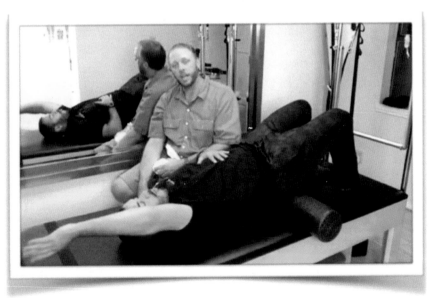

# Retrain The Brain—The Dunn Method

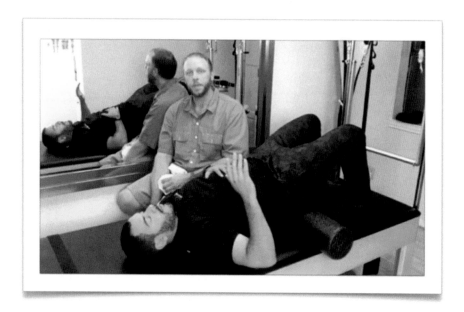

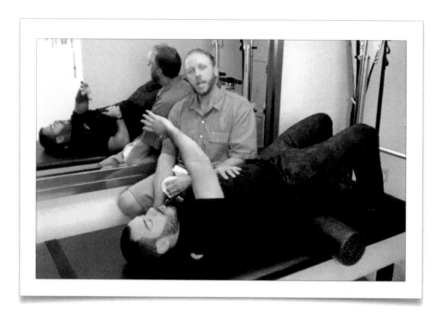

# Retrain The Brain—The Dunn Method

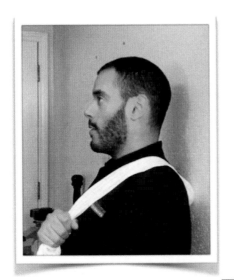

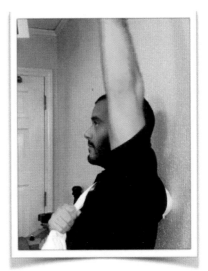

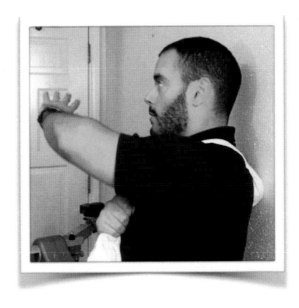

## Piriformis

The piriformis runs from the sacrum to the outer hip bone, deep under the gluteus maximus, or the buttock muscle. The piriformis is tight in many cases and can put pressure on the sciatic nerve. Many people stand with their feet turned out, also a sign of tightness in the piriformis.

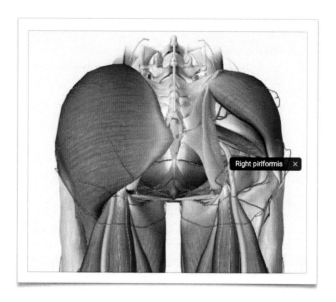

To release the left piriformis you are going to lay on your back with your left knee bent, foot flat on the ground. Place the tennis ball under your left buttock in the middle of your cheek. It may not be tender immediately, but when you let your left knee go out to the side, what I call the frog position, you will know then if the ball is in the correct spot. It will cause tension, pressure, and discomfort where the ball is. If it is not uncomfortable, you are in the wrong spot. Move it up, move it down, and move it in. Move it out half an inch or an inch until you find the painful spot. You may find multiple spots in the piriformis area that are tender and require some releasing.

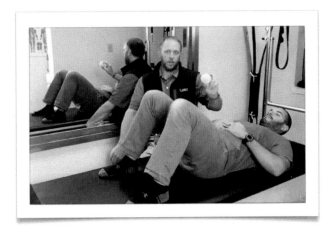

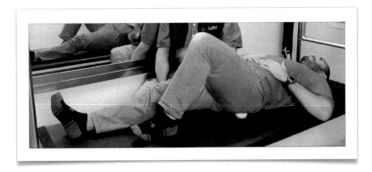

The second leg motion is to take the knee out to the side in the frog position. Next, slide your heel away from your body then back towards your body. Do not lift the foot off the ground as you are sliding it back and forth. Now repeat on the other side.

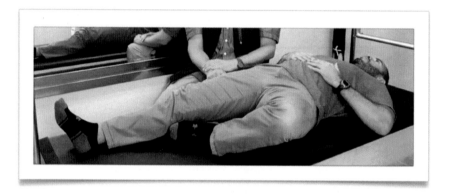

This concludes the first round of home exercises or what we call self- myofascial release. Grab your ball and get started now to release your psoas, iliacus, diaphragm, pectoralis minor, levator scapulae, and piriformis. Do both sides. It may be more painful on a side that you are not expecting. That is all for the release work. We are moving on to some basic core stabilization exercises.

To access the videos of each exercise, follow the link: https://pilatestothrive.com/backpain/

# Chapter Two

# Re-educating the Core with Static Exercise

It was January 2002 when Cheryl and I signed up to take our Pilates teacher training certification with Barbara Wintroub out in Santa Monica, California. On our first day of class, she did a postural assessment of each of us. It was shocking to discover that my posture had actually worsened since being in physical therapy school six years earlier.

At first, I questioned her, but she grabbed her digital camera and took a picture, hooked it up to her computer and showed me. Again, this was before smartphones with cameras everywhere. I had a flip phone at this time. Back to my posture. It was terrible. My head was forward, my thoracic spine was slouched, my hamstrings were shortened and my pelvis was pulled into a bad position. It was very shocking to see how bad my posture was. I had been treating patients for four years trying to teach them how to stand tall and sit tall and was wondering why they could not actually do it.

# Retrain The Brain—The Dunn Method

Well, I couldn't do it, so why should I expect to teach them to do it?

A light bulb went off in my head with my Pilates training and it had nothing to do with what I actually learned in Pilates. I was concerned with how bad my posture had worsened and I realized that I needed to improve my posture if I wanted to help my patients improve theirs.

Now that we have completed the release work it is time to re-educate the appropriate muscles. For this program to have the most benefit, the release work should be completed first, followed by the core re-education. This will create a new motor memory and basically re-educate old patterns that have been there for many, many years. This is the foundation of the strengthening we will build on. We call that the essential exercises.

In this second home exercise program, what you will need is a full, round, 36-inch by 6-inch foam roller. This three feet roller is round which allows you to lie on it. You can also use a half round roller but the full round roller is more effective and gives you many, many other options to do for other release type work. You also need two tennis balls and an old school blood pressure cuff, what I call a Joey Cuff.

Get your foam roller here...
(https://amzn.to/2zvNjWi)

Order your blood pressure cuff here...
(https://amzn.to/2KOaUpP)

## Lumbar Multifidus

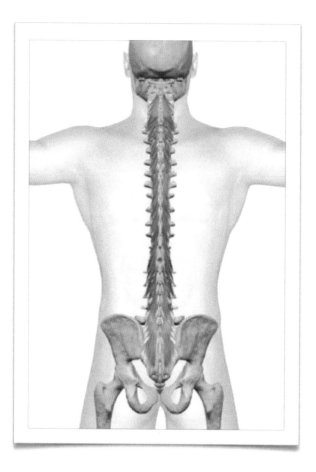

The multifidus is the antagonist to the hip flexors. With most people I treat, the psoas is super, super tight and the multifidus is very weak or not working. The multifidus will stabilize adjoining vertebrae and are important for control of the lumbar vertebrae during movement. The multifidus sits deep in the back of the spine and lies within the groove on the side of the spinous process of the vertebra. The Latin word for multifidus is as the following:

Multis" means many, and "findo" means cleave. When most people injure their lumbar spine for the first time, the lumbar multifidus stops working correctly. This muscle is hugely neglected for rehabilitating the lumbar spine. However, it's the most essential muscle for the lumbar spine to move efficiently inter segmentally, or at each lumbar segment.

How do we exercise the lumbar multifidus? We start with an exercise called the long bridge or the long bridge multifidus. You lay on your back with your legs relaxed and straight. Flex your feet, bringing your toes toward your nose. Bend your knees about six to eight inches, basically digging your heels down into the ground. The foam roller should fit under your knees as an example of the correct leg placement in space. In this position, you will push down into your heels and start to lift your buttocks, but do not actually lift your buttocks. Do not arch your back. Do not flatten your back. Do not move your pelvis. Just push into the heels, hold for five seconds, and then relax. The muscle is deep and close to your spine on either side of your spine. You will feel the multifidus bulging up at that moment as you push into your heels. Your hamstrings and glutes will also fire very firmly simultaneously. Complete this exercise for one minute, holding for five seconds at a time.

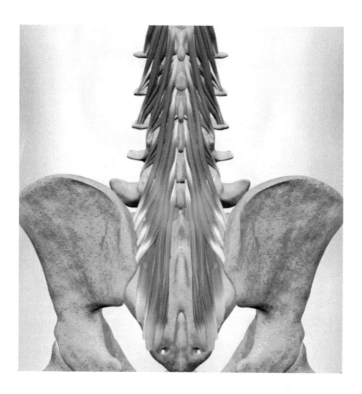

# Retrain The Brain—The Dunn Method

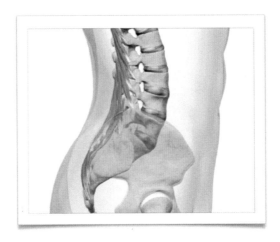

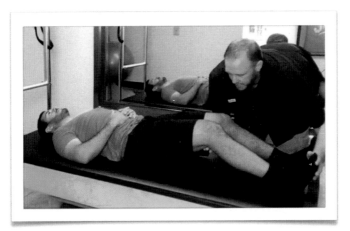

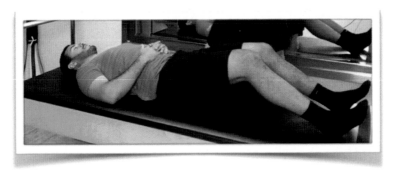

## The Respiratory Diaphragm

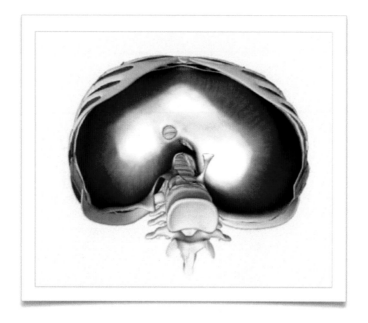

The diaphragm is shaped like a tent and runs from side to side and front to back under the ribs. It creates the shelf that the heart and lungs sit on as it separates the heart and lungs from the stomach, guts, intestines, et cetera. Its main purpose is for proper deep breathing. However, most people breath very shallow and only use a third of their lungs. This means the diaphragm doesn't work much at all, only the upper neck muscles and chest muscles. This is a major problem in our modern culture where people hold their breath when they exercise, hold their breath throughout the day, and have poor shallow breathing overall.

## Diaphragmatic Breathing

Lie on your back with your knees bent and your feet flat on the ground. Place your hands on the side of your ribs towards the bottom of your ribs with your fingers up towards the midline of your body and your thumbs towards the back. Take an inhale and push your hands away from each other with your ribs. On the exhale, bring your ribs closer together or back to the starting position. Inhale, expand your ribs and your hands should go apart. Exhale, and bring your hands back together with the movement coming from your ribs. Complete this exercise for one minute, inhaling and exhaling. This may cause a little dizziness or light-headedness as many people have not taken breathes this deeply in some time or ever.

# Retrain The Brain—The Dunn Method

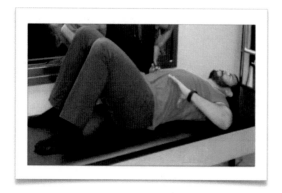

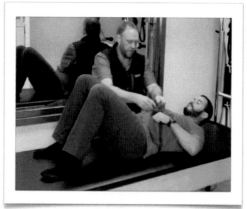

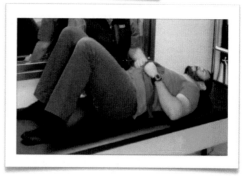

# Pelvic Floor

Think of the diaphragm as the top of the core. Now we will talk about the bottom of the core, the pelvic floor. There are two pelvic floor muscles, the levator ani, and the coccygeus.

These muscles form the flat, broad muscle of the pelvic floor, also known as the sling of the pelvic floor. There are also the sphincter muscles that control going to the bathroom, but we are not interested in those right now. Now I want to be clear. This is for men or women. The pelvic floor is not just for women. Men need to strengthen their pelvic floor as well and if they do, they will see a dramatic improvement in their back pain.

# Blood Pressure Cuff—Joey Cuff Exercise

You're going to sit on a firm chair, with a Joey Cuff placed directly between your two sits bones. You will then give a few pumps to the bulb on the end of the cord to inflate the blood pressure cuff and lift your pelvic floor.

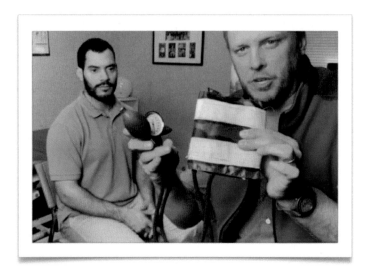

Retrain The Brain—The Dunn Method

Now you will look at the little glass piece that shows the readings with the numbers. Make sure you've pumped the ball up about 60 or 70 millimeters of Mercury. While sitting, rock your whole body back and forth and notice the needle on the gauge swing in a large direction up and down.

Now, sit still, find a good tall sitting position, and lift your pelvic floor, the sling. As you lift the pelvic floor, you should see the needle on the instrument pop up about two, three or four millimeters of Mercury, a small movement on the gauge. When you relax, the needle should pop back down. For many people, there will be very little movement of the needle at this point because of the weakness of the pelvic floor.

Retrain The Brain—The Dunn Method

Many of my clients have been instructed to stop the flow of urine at some point along the way. However, this is incorrect for what we are trying to accomplish with this exercise. If you stop the flow of urine, you're actually taking a sphincter muscle and doing something that it shouldn't do. A sphincter muscle is always tight and when it's time to go to the bathroom, we get it to relax and it opens and that's when we void. It is neurologically incorrect to try to get a sphincter muscle to close, as we only have the ability to open it. The sling should be lifting, not the sphincter tightening or closing. It's an inter-vaginal contraction with a lift of the pelvic floor, not at the sphincter. For men, we cue them to lift the boys.

# Retrain The Brain—The Dunn Method

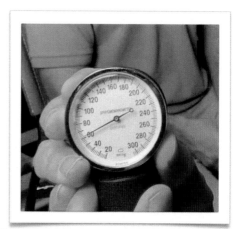

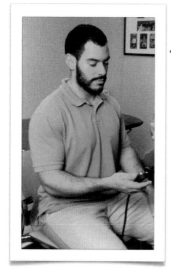

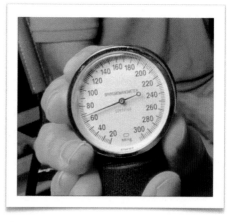

# Transversus Abdominis

The transversus abdominis (TA) is the deepest of the four abdominal muscles. The most superficial is the rectus abdominis, also known as "the six-pack". Then there's the external and internal oblique and then the deepest TA muscle.

The TA wraps around the body like a corset between the ribs and pelvis from front to back and to the side. The action of the TA is to compress the ribs and viscera and provide thoracic and pelvic stability. Most of my clients today are strong in their six-pack and one of their obliques, but usually weak in the deep abdominals.

# Co-Contraction

Now we will do an exercise we call the *co-contraction* or the deep abdominal breathing exercise. We call it a co-contraction be-cause it is the TA with the pelvic floor and the diaphragm all working together on the exhale. Lay on your back with your knees bent and your feet flat on the ground. Place your hands on your belly button and take an inhale and push your hands towards the ceiling with your abdominals. On the exhale, draw your belly button towards your spine, pulling your hands towards your spine. Most people will breathe into their chest at this point and have a hard time actually taking an inhale into their belly and making the belly rise towards the ceiling. Take your time with this and focus on inhaling, belly to the ceiling, then exhaling, belly button to the spine.

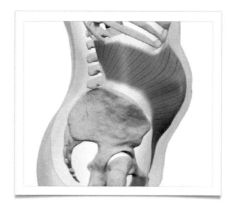

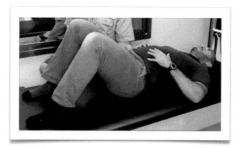

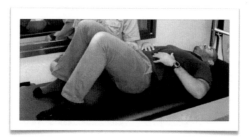

The majority of my clients must go into a slight posterior pelvic tilt at this point to get into an ideal spinal position. However, that is not the case for all of my clients.

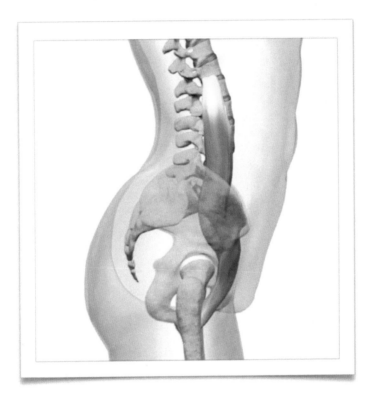

This is why a personal assessment is important. Learning these exercises and release work in person is the ideal way to start.

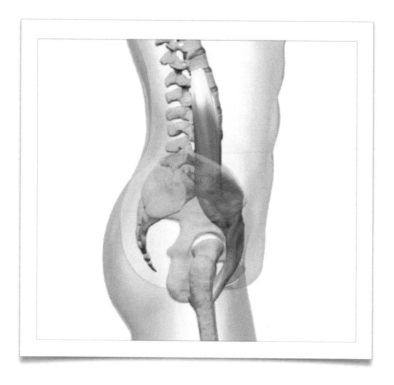

Now, I want you to take an inhale, belly button to the ceiling, and on the exhale, pull your belly button towards the spine. Flatten the lower back slightly, rocking your pelvis backward into what we call a slight pelvic tilt. This is also referenced as a north tilt or a 12 o'clock tilt. Again, most of my clients are stuck in a south tilt or a 6 o'clock tilt. Therefore, we are doing this 12 o'clock tilt or north tilt to get into a better spinal position.

This is the foundation for the exercises that we will do in the next chapter.

Retrain The Brain—The Dunn Method

To access the videos to each exercise, click here:
https://pilatestothrive.com/backpain/

# Chapter Three

# Being Mindful of The Basics: Let's Build to Dynamic Exercise.

A frequent question I get is how I got interested in **GYROTONIC®** exercise? I was exposed to Gyrotonic exercise at the Pilates studio where I worked in Santa Monica. However, back in 2002, it just didn't resonate with me. A year later, we were living in Sonoma, California. I was on a travel contract for physical therapy and Cheryl began her certification process at the studio where she was working. When we moved to Austin, we had a Gyrotonic tower sitting in our living room for a few months. I played around with it just enough to spike my curiosity. We opened CORE Therapy & Pilates six months later, and the Gyrotonic machine moved out of my living room and into the studio. This decreased my time to tinker with it.

After a few years of Cheryl teaching Pilates and Gyrotonic exercise, it was time to get a few new trainers to teach on this exercise tower. Cheryl arranged for a master trainer to come to Austin from California to teach a course.

Retrain The Brain—The Dunn Method

Five students signed up for the course, but the teacher required six. I was a little unsure, but I took it for the team and signed up as the sixth student to make the training happen. This allowed Cheryl to get help teaching on this new crazy looking machine.

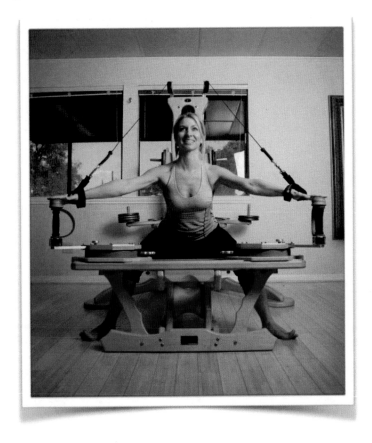

Pilates connected me with my core. Gyrotonic exercise connected me with my shoulder blades and actually taught me to sit and stand in a better posture.

Retrain The Brain—The Dunn Method

Dynamic exercise is defined as any exercise that involves joint movement. Typical exercises include squats, bicep curls, or push ups. It is very important to progress my clients from static exercises on your back to dynamic exercises. We begin the dynamic exercises lying on the foam roller. Next they complete the hands and knees in the quadruped position. They then progress to sitting with back support, then to sitting without back support and finally standing. The goal is to become aware and mindful of their pelvis, spine, scapula and head position with each exercise. We use Pilates and Gyrotonic exercises in private and group sessions to train our clients in this progression. The following outlines this progression in our home program.

Retrain The Brain—The Dunn Method

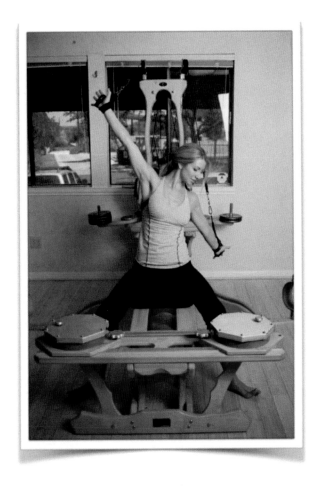

Sitting is the new smoking. Stand up desks are all the rage and many clients are getting stand up desks. Anyone with poor sitting posture is more likely to have poor standing posture. Basically, people must learn how to sit better and stand better. We find that the dynamic strengthening is a key to this.

For the third home exercise program, you will need a TheraBand (https://amzn.to/2re0V3Q) or TheraTube, red or green. You will need a full round foam roller, the 6-inch by 36-inch. You will need a ball of some size. The gold ball can work or a basketball or a volleyball. A Pilates ring (https://amzn.to/2LHq4A7) can also be used for this.

First, let's review the co-contraction because everything dynamically builds on the static co-contraction. Inhale and the belly rises to the ceiling. Exhale and the belly draws in towards the spine with a co-contraction of the core. This is done on your back with your knees bent and your feet flat on the ground.

## Ball Squeeze

Now we will do a ball squeeze to strengthen the inner thighs. Place a ball between your knees and squeeze as hard as you can. Did you notice your abdominals and pelvic floor contract? (Probably Not...)

Retrain The Brain—The Dunn Method

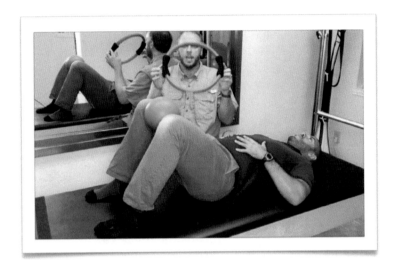

Let's focus. Pay attention. Co-contract first and then squeeze the ball. Inhale, belly to the ceiling. Exhale, belly to the floor. Lift the pelvic floor, tighten the deep abdominals, and then squeeze the ball between the knees at about 50-60%. This is about coordination and timing. This is not about brute strength. Squeeze the ball harder as the core control gets better and easier to find. Repeat for one minute.

# Retrain The Brain—The Dunn Method

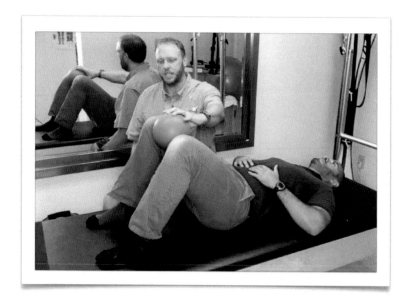

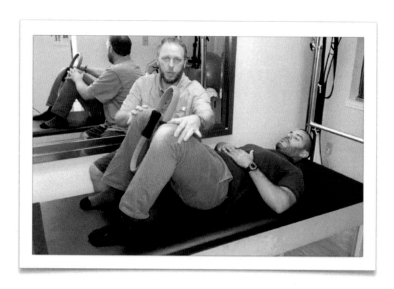

# Hip ABD/ER or Clam

Now we will take a TheraBand, and tie it in a knot to fit around your knees or we will use the Pilates Flex Ring around your knees. Inhale, belly to the ceiling. Exhale, belly to the floor. Open your legs pulling the resistive band or the Flex Ring apart. This is strengthening the outer muscles of your hips.

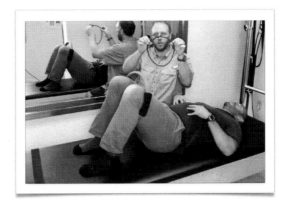

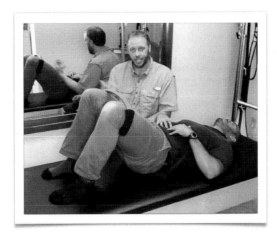

## **Alternating March or Tiny Steps**

Now we will strengthen those pesky hip flexors. Inhale, belly button to the ceiling. Exhale, belly button to the spine. Lift one leg in the air keeping the knee bent. The tiny step is on the exhale with the co-contraction. Think of floating the leg up gently. This is subtle, not forceful.

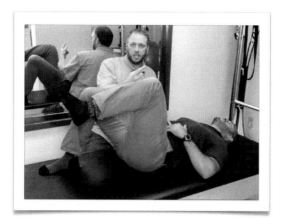

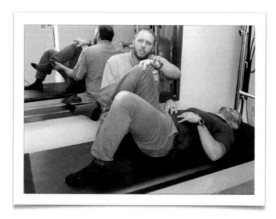

# Bridging

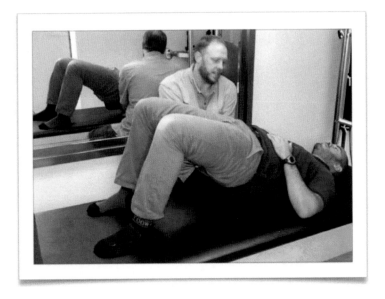

Now, we will do a bridge where we lift the rear end in the air on the exhale. Inhale to prepare. Exhale, and push through both feet and lift your bottom in the air. Inhale in the bridge position. Exhale, roll down one vertebra at a time, softening through the sternum and then the mid back. Lower your back until the pelvis is on the ground. To progress the bridge, lift on the exhale. Inhale, and straighten one leg in the air. Exhale to bring that leg back down to the ground. Inhale, and straighten the other leg to the air. Exhale, and bend that knee back down. Finally, lower down from the bridge one vertebra at a time as we already discussed. This is a much more challenging exercise and requires you to have a lot of pelvic stability. This means the pelvis should not be shifting back and forth as one leg is lifting.

We always tell our clients, "Your shoulder blades are not earrings. Get them out of your ears." So how do we actually get them out of our ears? How do we get our shoulders back and down? We use the latissimus dorsi (also known as the "lats"), the lower traps, and the rhomboids. The lats are large muscles that go from the front of the arm and armpit down to the back and pelvic area. The lower traps are the antagonists of the upper traps and are usually weak. They attach to the spine where the lumbar and thoracic spine come together with the diaphragm then ascend up to the shoulder blades. The lower traps help slide the shoulder blades down the ribcage. This is the opposite of what the upper traps do. They elevate the shoulder blades up towards the ears.

Lastly, we will talk about the rhomboid major and rhomboid minor, which we will refer to as the rhomboids. The rhomboids squeeze the shoulder blades together. This is the opposite of what the pectoral minor does to pull the shoulder blades forward. These muscles are located deep beneath the trapezoids and attach from the spine to the medial border of the shoulder blades. We can say that these shoulder blade muscles have been locked long or locked in a stretched position. The antagonist muscles are locked short and tight.

## Scapula Setting

To strengthen the shoulder blade muscles, we will do an exercise called the scapula setting exercise. Lay on your foam roller long ways from your buttocks to your head with your knees bent and your arms out to the side.

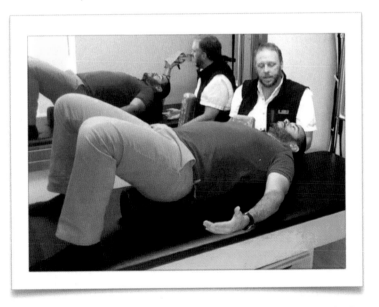

Before we do any strengthening of the shoulder blades, let's open the chest with a quick review of the co-contraction of your deep abdominals, pelvic floor, and diaphragm for 3-5

minutes. Now, grab the two tennis balls and place them under each hand with your elbows straight and the balls next to your sides (the pictures and video will not show the tennis balls, they are not required but help coordinate this exercise better). Slide your shoulder blades up towards your ears and down towards your pelvis. Keeping your elbows straight, roll with your hands up and down on the tennis balls.

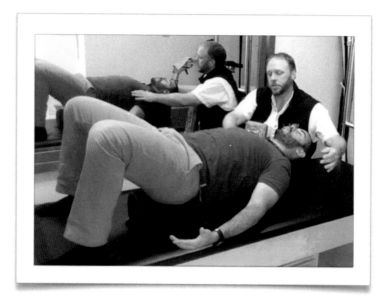

Now let's add in the breathing. Inhale, and shrug your shoulders up towards your ears. Keep those elbows straight. Exhale to slide the shoulders down towards your pant pockets. Don't forget your abdominals. Inhale, belly button to the ceiling, shoulder blades to the ears. Exhale, belly button to the spine. Engage the core, sliding the shoulder blades down the spine, setting the scapula. Inhale then exhale. We're now putting it all together. Inhale, scapulae elevate. Exhale, scapulae depress. This is where we coordinate the lumbar stabilization with scapula stabilization and what we call a co-contraction with scapula setting.

## Foam Roller Lat Pull

Now, we will add some resistance with the TheraBand and do what's called a "lat pull." Secure the TheraBand between the door and a doorknob with a knot by opening the door and then shutting the knot on the other side of the door. The TheraBand will be placed at the height of the door handle. Place the foam roller about a foot away from the door and lay on it with your head towards the door.

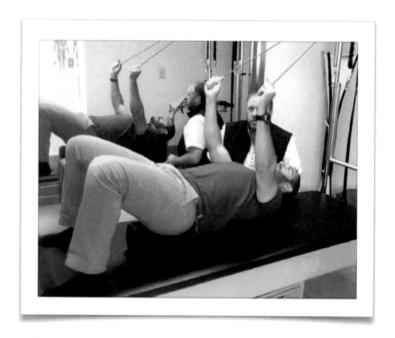

Lie on the foam roller, and reach up and grab the two ends of the TheraBand. Lift your arms to the ceiling with your elbows straight. Inhale, stay in that position. Exhale, co-

contract, bring your shoulder blades back and down. Pull both hands down to the sides.

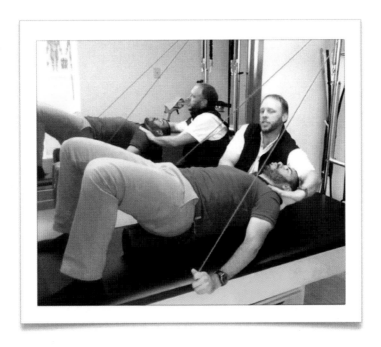

Inhale as your arms float back up. Exhale, pull down. Coordinating the lumbar and scapula stabilization concepts takes a lot of concentration.

## Foam Roller Horizontal ABD

Remove the TheraBand from the doorframe and grab it in your hands as you're on the roller again. Have your palms up, elbows straight, arms in front of you. Inhale to prepare. As you exhale and co-contract, pull the band apart by squeezing the shoulder blades together, opening your chest. As you inhale, your hands come back to the ceiling. As you exhale, pull apart. We call this horizontal abduction.

# Retrain The Brain—The Dunn Method

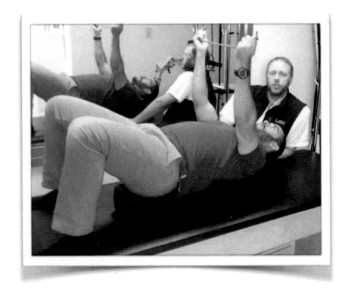

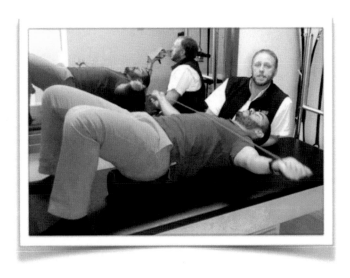

## Foam Roller Rotator Cuff

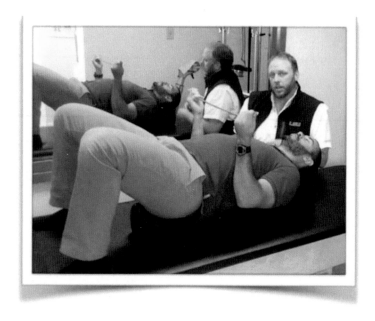

Now, we will strengthen the rotator cuff with something we call horizontal external rotation. Bend your elbows and place them at your side palms facing up. Keep your elbows at your side and pull the resistive band apart on the exhale. Inhale return to the starting position. Exhale as you co-contract and pull the resistance band. Notice a common theme here? The breathing, co-contraction, the abdominals, pelvic floor, low back position, and shoulder blade position are very important for every exercise.

# Retrain The Brain—The Dunn Method

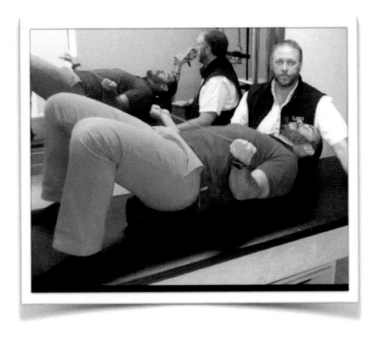

## Quadruped Co-Contraction

Now, we will go to a hands and knees position called quadruped. First, we will do the co-contraction. As you inhale, the belly is going towards the floor and as you exhale, you're pulling your belly button away from the floor towards your spine. Inhale, the belly sags. Exhale, co-contact, and pull up towards the spine.

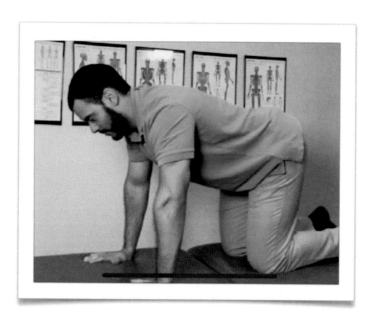

## Quadruped Leg Lifts

Now, we will add alternating hip extension. Inhale to prepare and then exhale, co-contract. Extend one leg in the air with the knee straight, keeping it parallel to the floor. As you inhale, return that leg back to the ground. On the next exhale, alternate and extend the opposite leg. The goal is to keep the pelvis stable and the spine still as you are extending the legs. Be mindful of your back and down shoulder blade position. Do not hyperextend your elbows.

# Retrain The Brain—The Dunn Method

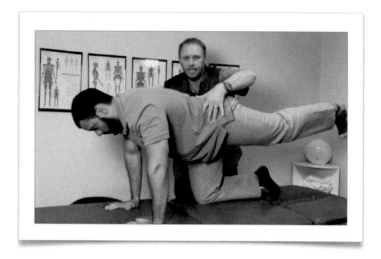

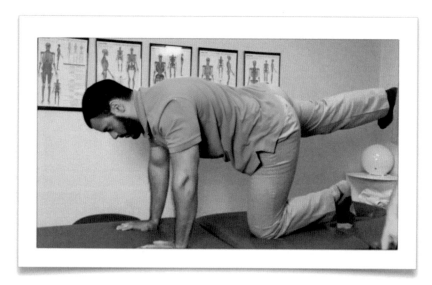

## Quadruped Arm Lifts

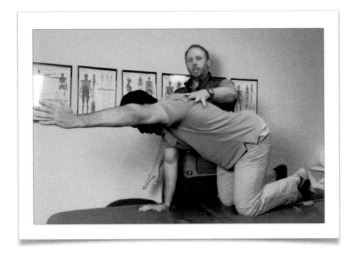

Now, we will lift the arms on the exhale. Inhale, belly to the floor. Exhale, and pull the belly up. Set the shoulder blade back and down as you lift one arm up in front, parallel to the floor. Inhale, return the hand to the floor and exhale, bring the opposite arm up. Focus and take your time with this exercise.

# Retrain The Brain—The Dunn Method

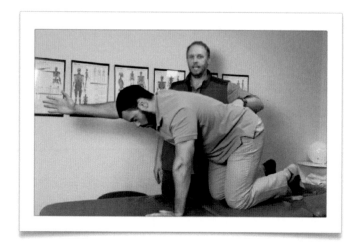

## Quadruped Alternating Arm and Leg Lifts

The final step in quadruped is the most challenging. Alternate lifting the opposite arm and leg. Lift the right leg and left arm at the same time on the exhale. Maintain a strong and stable spine. Inhale and lower the arm and leg back to quadruped. Lift the left leg and right arm as you stabilize the spine and shoulder blades. Repeat for one minute.

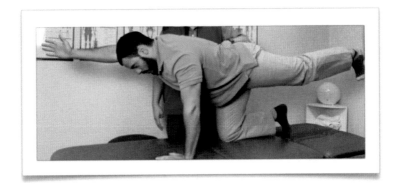

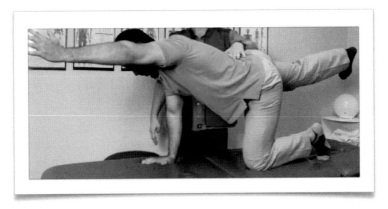

## Sitting Foam Roller Lat Pull

We now move to sitting in a chair with a pool noodle or the foam roller behind our back. This allows you to open the chest and move the shoulder blades. Place the chair facing the door about 2 feet from the door. Take the TheraBand with a knot in it and attach it above the door between the door and the doorframe. Sitting in the chair, arms straight in front of you, inhale without moving. Exhale, pulling straight down by your side. Maintain your co-contraction. Keep your shoulder blades back and down. This is the exact same thing you were doing on the foam roller, but now you're sitting and the load of the spine is very different. Repeat all of these for a minute.

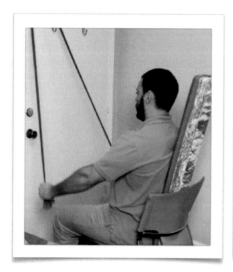
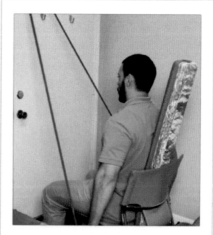

## Sitting Foam Roller Rows

We will now do a rowing motion. Move the band down between the door and the doorframe at the height of the doorknob. Inhale to prepare. Exhale and bend your elbows as you pull the band towards your lower ribs.

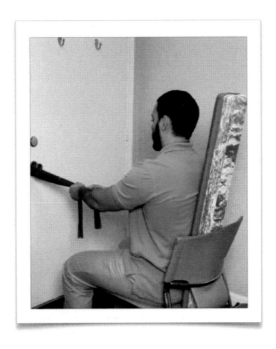

Maintain your co-contraction as you row. Inhale, and straighten the elbows towards the door. Exhale to pull the resistance band toward you while opening the chest. Repeat exercise for one minute.

# Retrain The Brain—The Dunn Method

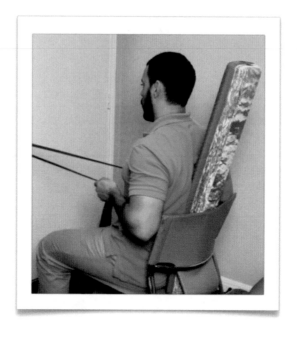

## Sitting Lat Pull and Rows

Now you will repeat those same two exercises without the back support. Scoot up to the front of the chair. Find that good spine position without feedback from the foam roller or pool noodle. This is a challenging exercise. Several weeks of practicing the previous exercises with back support may be necessary to achieve success.

# Retrain The Brain—The Dunn Method

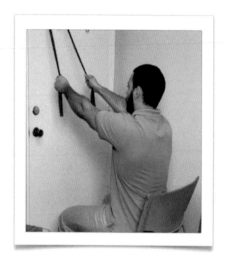

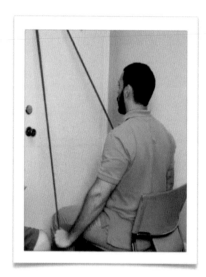

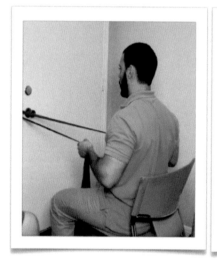

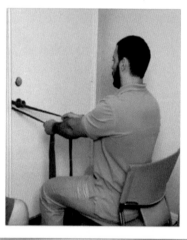

## Standing Co-Contraction

The last progression for this chapter is standing. In standing, lift the toes, but not the toe balls. Shift your weight back into your heels. This automatically puts your pelvis and lumbar spine in a better position.

Now, create a co-contraction while you open your chest and lengthen your spine out of the crown of your head. Standing is a very active process if you're doing it right. With practice of this routine, your standing will become better and better. That stand-up desk (https://amzn.to/2KLTFFy) (https://amzn.to/2Slp7wR) will make a lot of sense once you've gone through this strengthening program.

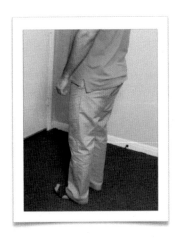
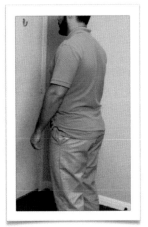

## Standing Lat Pull

Now, let's grab the theraband again and repeat the lat pull and rowing exercise while standing. Attach the TheraBand above the door for the lat pull. Stand about 3 feet away from the door, facing the door. Grab the TheraBand on both ends and keep your arms straight. Inhale to prepare. Exhale, lift the toes, co-contract, with shoulders back and down as you pull the TheraBand down by your side. Inhale as you float your arms back to the starting position, releasing the tension on the resistance band. Exhale as you repeat all the steps. Be mindful.

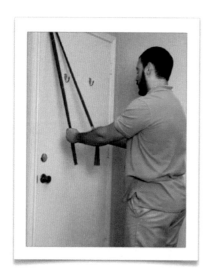 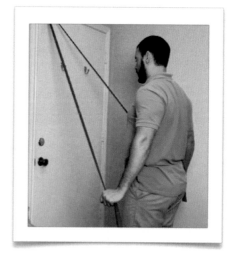

## Standing Row

Rowing is the same as described in sitting, but now you are standing with great focus and awareness. Inhale to prepare. Exhale and pull the resistance band towards your lower ribs. Bend your elbows and open your chest. Do not arch your back. Keep that co-contraction strong.

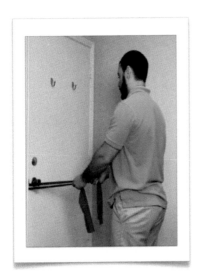 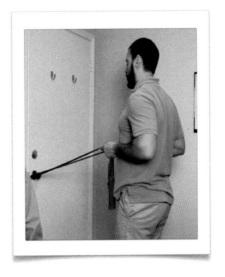

This concludes this chapter and this round of new exercises.

To access the videos of each exercise, follow the link:

https://pilatestothrive.com/backpain/

# Chapter Four

# Applying Core Strength to your Day to Day Life, Sports, and Recreation

When Cheryl and I signed up to do our Pilates teacher training, we had also just signed up to do a marathon training to raise money for the stroke association. Both programs started in January of 2002. As we started learning Pilates and applying Pilates to our day-to-day life, I wanted to be able to apply the breathing to my walking marathon training. Each month my breathing got better, my strength got better, my posture improved with training, and so did my day-to-day activities, like lifting my 75# boxer.

We had a practice marathon on Cinco de Mayo in Pacific Palisades, California. It was a gorgeous morning walking on the coast overlooking the Pacific Ocean. This was also a distraction as I had a hard time keeping my breathing and my focus while performing my walk. I would breathe, inhale, exhale, keeping my abdominals engaged on the exhale, keeping my shoulders in a good position. I would get into that for several minutes and then suddenly I'd see a whale out in the ocean and I would lose it all. I would start slacking and walking lethargically. Then I would remember, because of the new awareness that I had, and I would self-correct my posture and get back into my breathing and my rhythm.

I was doing half marathons for this and for the next one, while Cheryl was doing marathons. So, the numbers I reference are involved with my half marathons. Then on June 23rd, we went to complete a half marathon and marathon in Hawaii on the big island, on the Iron Man Course. It was very hot compared to the training we were used to in Los Angeles. And humid, humid, humid. But something had clicked from Cinco de Mayo to the middle of June. It wasn't that I had gotten better walking, or that I'd gotten stronger, but my awareness had improved and I was able to breathe, and focus, and keep my intention on good posture and good form the entire half marathon. No distractions, no lack of focus, I was able to improve my time by 15 minutes over a seven-week period, by only breathing and paying attention, and applying everything that I had learned over the previous six months with Pilates. That's when I knew I had to teach Pilates to all my clients, and that it could change things for them for the better in so many ways.

At the same time in my life, I was playing softball on four or five different teams in Los Angeles. Most were competitive, and one team was pretty pathetic. But I noticed that I was applying my Pilates breath, and I was exhaling as I swung the bat to strike the softball. My core was also engaged. I had been playing baseball and softball since I was five years old, and here I was at 29 years old hitting the ball further and harder than I ever had in my life. I attribute this to my core strength and my new breathing technique applied to my softball swing. Then I noticed my snowboarding improving, my ability to play basketball, and all things recreationally were better than they had been over the previous 10 years.

I hope my story resonates with you. So, everything so far is to get to this point, to apply the mental training, the awareness training to our day to day activities, our recreation and our sports. Whether it's sitting at the computer, working out at the gym, playing golf or tennis, walking the dog, lifting a box at the house, or getting laundry out of the dryer.

Retrain The Brain—The Dunn Method

We will break the next home exercise program into two parts. The first part is the dowel program, and the second part is what we're going to call basic Pilates mat work. You will need a three-foot, wooden or plastic dowel, about the size of a broomstick, or you can use a broomstick.

Wooden dowels can be purchased at the link...

(https://amzn.to/2SiDUbt)

## Dowel Standing Exercise

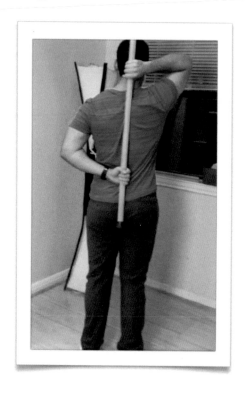

In standing, place the dowel behind your back. You're going to use both hands to hold the dowel with one hand above your head, and one hand holding the dowel in the small of your back. Place the back of your hand towards the lower back. Inhale to prepare, exhale and lift your toes, keeping the toe balls on the ground. Lean slightly back on your heels lifting your spine by keeping your lower back, mid back, and head in contact with the dowel as best as possible. This creates length and decompression of your spine. Inhale relax, and you will notice your weight shift forward slightly. Exhale, lift your toes, lean back into the heels, and engage the back line of your glutes and hamstring while lengthening your spine. Repeat for one minute, inhaling and exhaling.

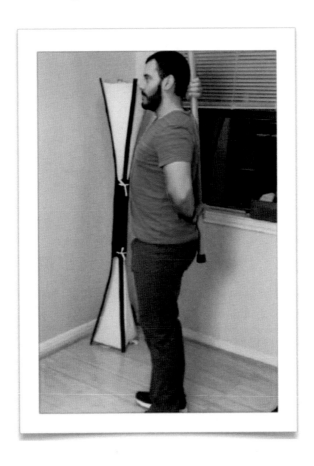

## Dowel Hip Hinge

Standing with your feet shoulder-width apart and the dowel behind your back as previously described. Inhale to prepare. Exhale, lift your toes which creates an arch lift in the foot. Lengthen your spine as you bend your knees about 45 degrees and reach your butt away from your head as your chest and head go forward over your toes. Keep your spine in contact with the dowel as best as possible. Inhale as you return to standing, exhale as you perform the hip hinge and repeat. This is the prerequisite to go from standing to sitting or to reverse it and go from sitting to standing. Whether it's down to a chair, a toilet, or in and out of a car, you can progress the hip hinge by standing and going all the way down to touch your rear on the seat. Maintaining the length in your spine and the co-contraction of your deep abdominals and pelvic floor.

# Retrain The Brain—The Dunn Method

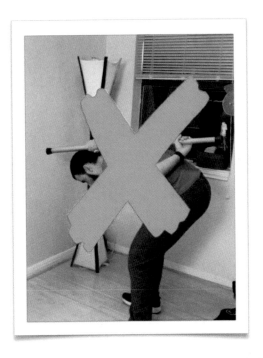

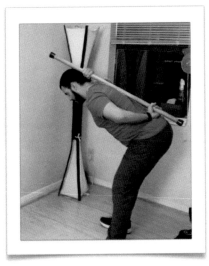

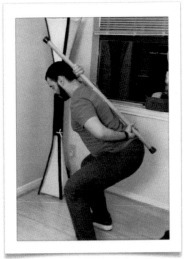

# Dowel Plié

Stand with your heels together and your toes, knees and hips slightly turned out with the dowel behind your spine. With this exercise, your knees will bend and your heels will stay together and you will slide your buttocks towards your heels. You will not be leaning forward. It's as if you are sliding up and down on a pole with your spine. Inhale to prepare. Exhale, lift the toes, lengthen the spine and bend the knees to about 30 degrees. Inhale, return to standing tall, exhale, and repeat. Repeat this exercise for one minute, inhaling and exhaling the entire time. Maintain length through the spine on every exhale.

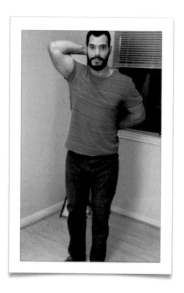 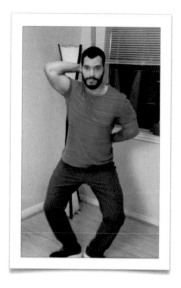

## Lunge Series

To set up, Place your right foot forward with your knee straight and your foot flat on the ground. Place your left leg behind you with your knee straight and up on your toes with your heel off the ground. Keep your back heel in line with your knee and hip, not turned out to the side.

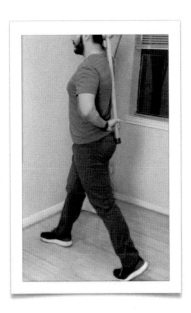
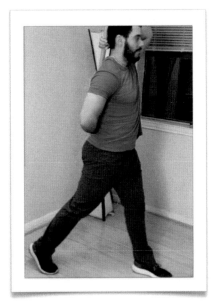

## Step 1: Front Knee Bend

Maintain the lunge set up position with the dowel behind your back, and bend the front knee five to ten degrees without losing the position of the pelvis or spine, or length of the spine. Inhale to prepare. Exhale, and bend the knee around ten degrees, while maintaining everything in line. Repeat for one minute. Switch the legs and put the left leg forward with the right leg back and repeat.

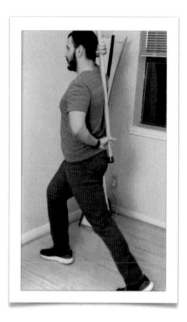 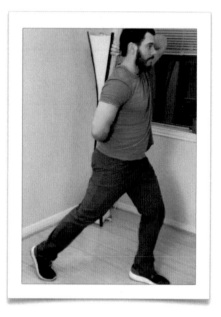

## Step 2: Back Knee Bend

With the right leg forward and the left leg backward, extend both knees with the left heel off the ground on the left tippy toes. Inhale to prepare. Exhale, and maintain the length in the spine using the dowel for feedback and bend the back knee 10 to 15 degrees without losing the position of the pelvis or the spine. Continue for 1 minute with breathing and repeat on the other side.

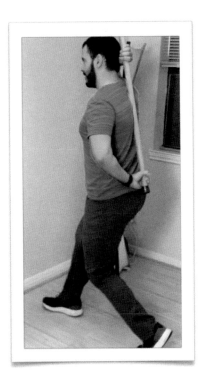 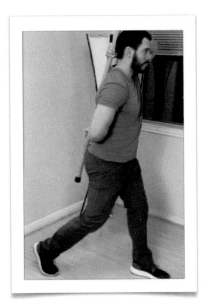

## Step 3: Mini Lunge

Partially bend both knees. With the right leg forward and the left leg back, extend both knees with the left heel off the ground on the left tippy toes.

Bend both knees slightly on the exhale. Maintain the length of the spine with feedback from the dowel. Return to the starting position on the inhale. Exhale, and lower down into the mini lunge. Repeat for one minute, and then switch legs and repeat for one minute.

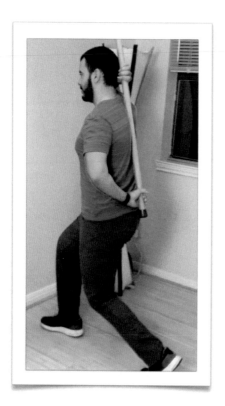
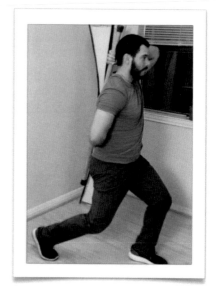

## Step 4: Full Lunge

Now, we are going to progress to the last exercise bending both knees and doing a full lunge. We are going to exhale on the way down and on the way up. With the right leg forward and the left leg back, inhale to prepare.

Exhale, and lengthen the spine and lower down all the way until the left knee is on the ground, right knee is bent around 90 degrees. Inhale in the full lunge, and exhale to co-

contract your abdominals, lengthen your spine as you return back to the starting position.

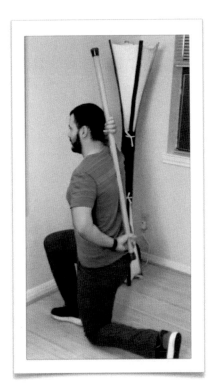
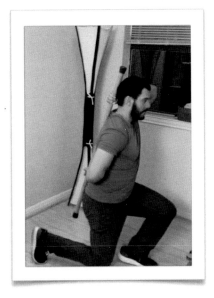

This concludes the dowel program, and we will now go into a basic Pilates mat program.

To access the videos of each exercise, follow the link: https://pilatestothrive.com/backpain/

# Chapter 5

# Pilates Workbook

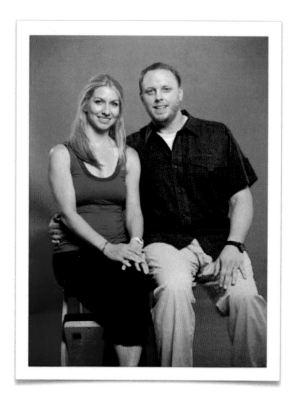

I am Cheryl Dunn, co-owner of CORE Therapy & Pilates. I want to talk to you a little bit about how I got into teaching Pilates and Gyrotonic exercise, the process and the steps that I took to get to where I am today. I was working a desk job and going to the gym every evening and enjoying the movement. I thought, you know I should get paid to do these classes and exercise because I enjoy it and I'm here anyway. So I went through a personal training certification through ACE to be able to do that and was able to teach a few classes here and there. Then I started hearing about Pilates a lot and so I started taking some Pilates classes and found some books on it and was doing a little bit here and there. And then Stephen comes to me and asked… "What's Pilates?"

So I tell him what I know and how I like it and what it's doing for me. He then got the opportunity to go through a Pilates teacher training, and I was thinking this is something to do. We talked to the Instructor, and she said of course. I went through the training with him and was able to start teaching Pilates. I eventually decided to teach Pilates exclusively.

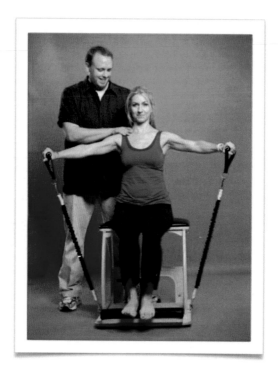

I worked with Stephen part-time in Burbank and part-time for a chiropractor in Beverly Hills. I was teaching their patients Pilates and helping them with what I knew. The major motivator was to show how much Pilates has helped me. Then Stephen and I got married and we moved to Sonoma.

The studio I worked at offered Gyrotonic exercise, and I was able to go through my Gyrotonic teacher training program. That led me to teaching both Pilates and Gyrotonic exercise. I really loved the two systems and how they meshed together and complemented each other. This led me to where I am today, opening up and running our own studio.

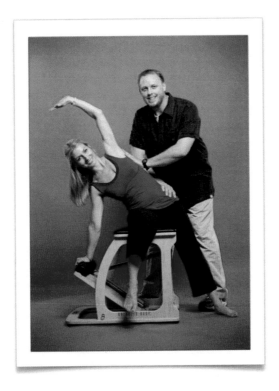

I have two boys now, so I don't work all day. I take them to school in the morning then work from 9:00 to 2:00 so that I can be there every afternoon to pick them up from school. I run them around and do all the things that need to happen in order to keep up with all their activities. I'm able to adjust my schedule to their schedules because their schedules have changed as they've grown up. When they were babies it was different. I had a different schedule. When they were in preschool, I worked a little less. Now that they're in school, so I can work and continue to provide people with two exercise modalities that can really help them. I get to teach people how much I enjoy it and what they can get from it. I have stayed strong and active and continue to do things with my kids and my family as I age. I enjoy the flexibility my work affords me. That's my story and how I got to where I am today.

Now, I want to teach you some Pilates exercises.

When someone is re-introducing movement into their life after an episode of back pain, they want to do it with caution and mindfulness. There are 6 main principles of Pilates that need to be addressed in every exercise. Listed below are the 6 Principles, and a list of questions to ask yourself to insure you are implementing each principle:

1. **Centering**—Where am I moving from? (i.e. Did I initiate this movement from my feet or do I initiate this from my core?)
2. **Breathing**—Is my breath supporting me or hindering me?
3. **Precision**—Is my body moving where and how it's supposed to be?

4. **Control**–Could I stop without jerking in any part of this exercise?
5. **Concentration**–Am I present or is my mind elsewhere?
6. **Dynamic Movement**–Am I enjoying the movement? (i.e. Too much control inhibits the movement.)

# PREPERATION FOR PILATES MAT WORK

## PELVIC CLOCKS

**Objective:** Bring awareness to the deep abdominals and pelvic mobility. This exercise will also release the lumbar spine and teach rotation initiated in the pelvis and hip joint.

**Starting Position:** Supine on your back. Lay on your back with your knees bent and feet flat on the floor. Place your arms next to you with your palms on the floor.

## Movement for 12 o'clock and 6 o'clock:

- Inhale to prepare.
- Exhale, and co-contract while curling the pubic bone towards the belly button (12 o'clock). The weight will come off of the tailbone and the PSIS (Posterior Superior Iliac Spine) will become heavy into the floor as you tilt your pelvis posteriorly. The PSIS is the bony part of the SI joint where the sacrum and ilium bones connect. This area is known by the two dimples on either side of the top of the sacrum.
- Inhale, and allow the pelvis to relax back into your resting position.

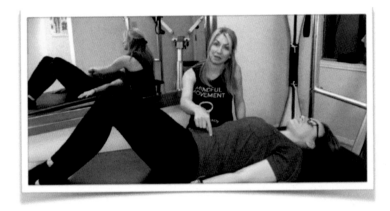

- Exhale, and co-contract while making the tailbone heavy and allowing the PSIS to come off the floor (6 o'clock) as you tilt your pelvis forward.

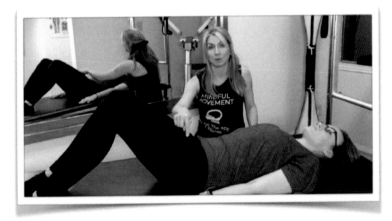

- Inhale, and allow the pelvis to relax back into a neutral position.
- Repeat in both directions, 6 o'clock and 12 o'clock, for 4 to 5 times.

## Movement for 3 o'clock and 9 o'clock:

- Inhale to prepare.
- Exhale, and co-contract while drawing the (L) PSIS down to the floor while the (R) PSIS rises towards the ceiling (3 o'clock).

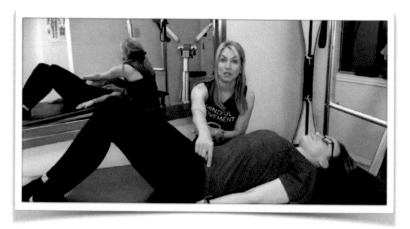

- Inhale while allowing the pelvis to relax back into your resting position.
- Exhale, and co-contract while drawing the (R) PSIS down to the floor while the (L) PSIS rises towards the ceiling (9 o'clock).

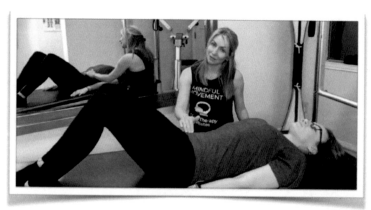

- Inhale while allowing the pelvis to relax back into your resting position.
- Repeat in both directions, 3 o'clock and 9 o'clock, for 4 to 5 times.

## Around the World

- Breathe continuously through this exercise while maintaining the co-contraction the whole time.
- Begin moving the pelvis to 12 o'clock, 3 o'clock, 6 o'clock and then 9 o'clock. The pelvis is moving in a circular motion.
- Do this for 4-5 times in both directions, clockwise and counterclockwise.

# SCAPULAR STABILITY AND MOBILITY

## Coronal Scapula Circles

**Objective:** Awareness of the shoulder blades (scapulae) moving on the ribcage.

**Starting Position:** Sit upright on top of the sits bones with the spine lifted, ribcage and head directly over the pelvis, shoulders abducted to the side at 90 degrees, and elbows bent to 90 degrees in the scapular plane.

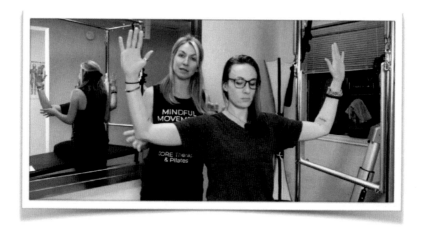

**Movement Sequence:**

- Inhale, and squeeze the shoulder blades together (adduct), and elevate the scapulae.

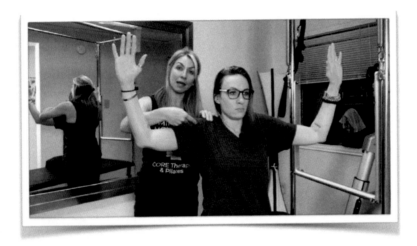

- Exhale to spread the blades apart (abduct) and then lower them.
- Repeat this motion for 4 to 5 times.

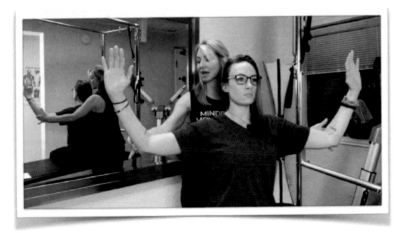

## Scapular Reaches

**Objective:** Awareness of the shoulder (humeral head) and scapula in a neutral position, movement awareness of the shoulder rotating in and out (internal and external rotation), and scapular movement on the ribcage.

**Starting Position:** Supine Home Position with hands raised above your chest, fingertips reaching up to the ceiling and your palms facing each other.

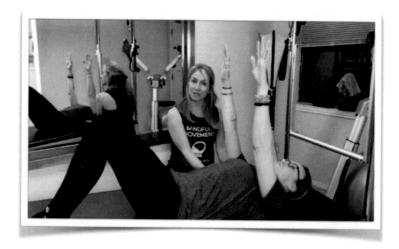

- Inhale, and reach the right arm toward the ceiling with scapula wide on the back, and externally rotate the arm. Your pinky fingers will rotate towards your midline, palms up.

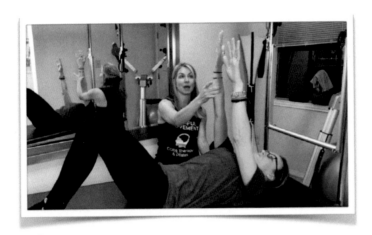

## Movement Sequence:

- Exhale to internally rotate right arm as if you are unscrewing a light bulb, as your shoulder blade returns to the starting position.
- Repeat the entire movement on the left arm.

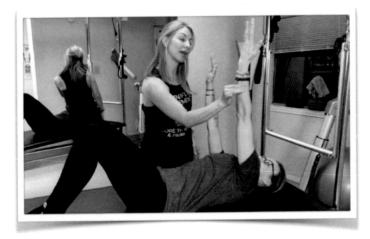

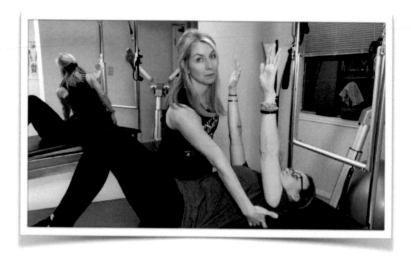

- Alternate this movement while maintaining contact with the floor with the scapula anchored.

# HEAD MOVEMENT

## Skull Bowl

**Objective:** To improve head placement on the spine and feel the release of the suboccipital muscles at the base of the skull.

**Starting Position:** Supine on your back.

**Movement Sequence:**

- Inhale to prepare.
- Exhale, and gently lengthen the head and tail away from each other. There is a slight chin tuck happening here on the exhale.

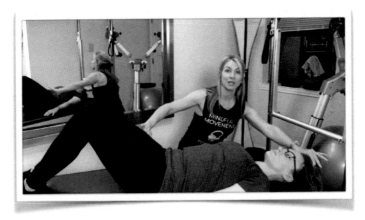

- Continue to breathe in a rhythmic breath, and nod the head *"YES"*. The cervical spine is moving in extension and flexion. Repeat for 4 to 5 times.

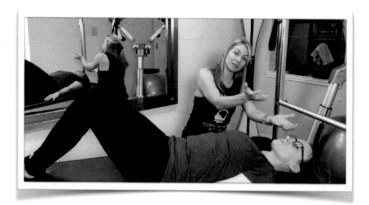

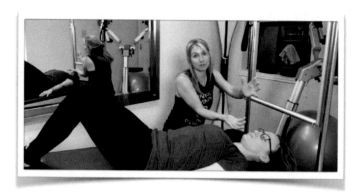

- Continue with the rhythmic breath nod the head saying *"NO"*. The cervical spine is now rotating side to side. Repeat for 4 to 5 times.

# Retrain The Brain—The Dunn Method

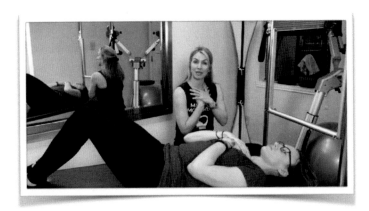

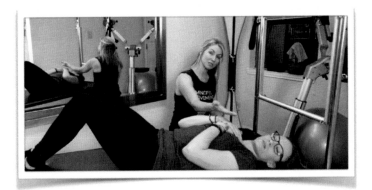

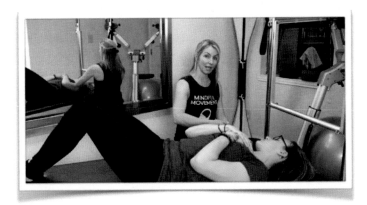

- Continue with the rhythmic breath, and trace a small circle with the nose.

# Head Float

**Objective:** Preparation for Pilates exercises that begin with neck flexion; strengthening the deep neck flexors, the deep abdominals and obliques.

**Starting Position:** Supine home position with hands clasped behind the neck; the pinky fingers under the occiput, and the elbows/shoulders relaxed.

**Movement Sequence:**

- Inhale to prepare.
- Exhale, and co-contract and begin the skull bowl flexion. Curl around the cervical spine, and continue to curl up sequentially to your scapular anchor points (the lower tips).

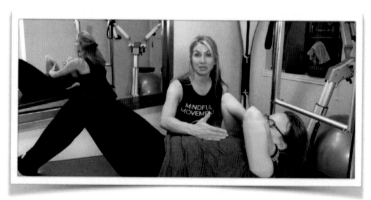

## Retrain The Brain—The Dunn Method

- Hold the position for 3 full breaths. Then, exhale, and deepen the co-contraction.
- On the last exhale, and sequentially roll back to the home position. Repeat this exercise for 4-5 times.

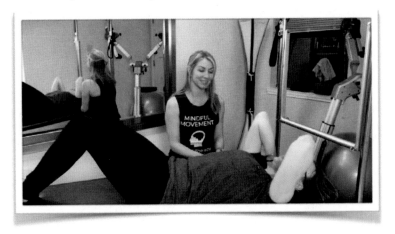

# PILATES MAT EXERCISES

Perform 4-5 reps of each with focus on form and breathing properly.

## The Roll Up

**Starting Position:** Lie on your back with your hands overhead. The arms can only go over the head as far as you can keep your lower back rib attached to the floor. Your arms may not be touching the floor.

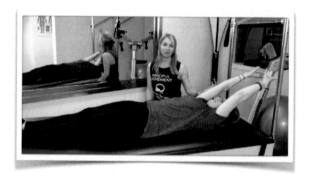

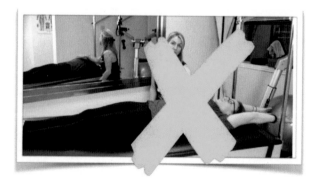

**Movement Sequence:**

- Inhale, and flex your feet, co-contract and reach the arms to the ceiling.
- Exhale, and peel the head and upper body off of the mat. Continue peeling your torso off the mat until you are sitting up on your sits bones. The upper body is curved over and reaching toward the feet as if you are wrapping your body over a giant beach ball.

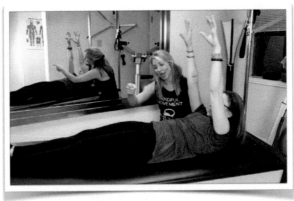

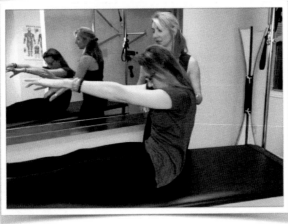

Retrain The Brain—The Dunn Method

- Inhale, and expand the back of the ribs while still reaching over your imaginary beach ball.

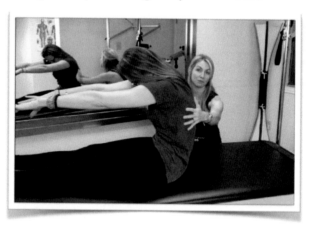

- Exhale, co-contract, and tuck your tailbone under while reaching your sits bones towards your heels and begin rolling down. Maintain the curve in your spine, and complete the roll down by reaching the arms over your head returning to the starting position.

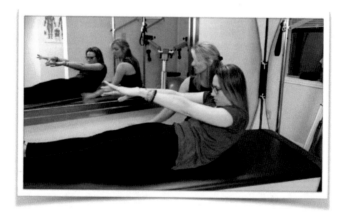

**Need Extra Help:** Place a rolled up hand towel at the small of your back. Push your spine into the towel as you are rolling up and down.

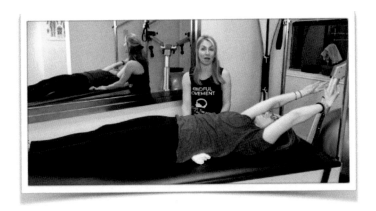

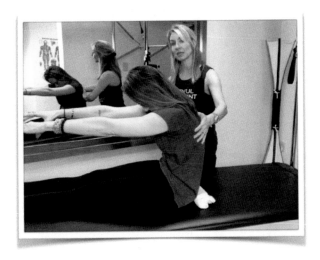

**Precautions:** Bend your knees slightly if you are unable to get your back flat on the floor to start.

## Rolling Like A Ball

**Starting Position:** Sit up on top of the sits bones, knees tucked into the body and arms wrapped around your shin bones. Take your feet off the floor while balancing between the sits bones and tailbone. Relax the shoulders away from the ears, keep the elbows wide and focus your eyes at your mid thigh. Keep the upper body rounded.

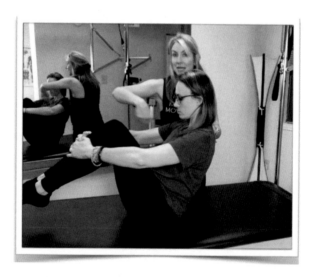

**Movement Sequence:**

- Inhale, co-contract, and pull the abdominals towards the spine to begin rolling backwards. Roll only to the tip of the shoulder blades.

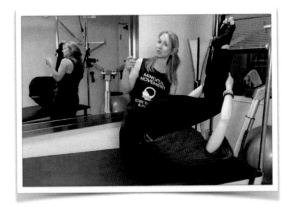

- Exhale, and squeeze the abdominals to begin rolling back up to your starting position. Balance in this position before beginning again.

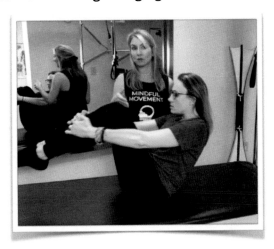

**Need Extra Help:** Place the hands on the back of your thighs rather than your shin bones. Be sure and push your thigh into hands and pull back with your hands at the same time. For a bony sacrum, place a folded towel on each side of the sacrum to create a channel for your sacrum to roll.

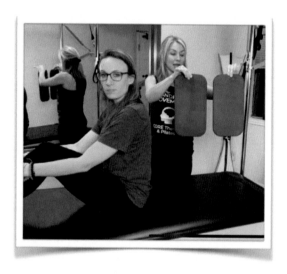

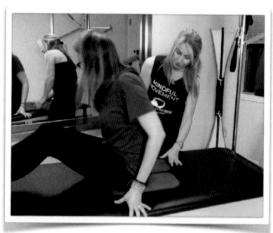

**Precautions:** If you strike the ground firmly and are unable to round your lower back enough to perform this exercise, release your hip flexors first and then try again.

Have you noted any difference after performing the psoas and iliacus release?

# Swan

**Starting Position:** Lie on your stomach with your elbows bent and palms on the mat next to your shoulders. Your legs are as close together as possible for the comfort of your lower back.

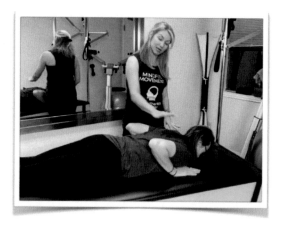

**Movement Sequence:**

- Inhale, co-contract, and slide the shoulder blades down the back. Press into the palms while floating the head off the mat. Continue to extend your spine while pressing the top of the thighs into the mat. Rise up only as far as the lower back is comfortable. Keep the head in line with the spine.

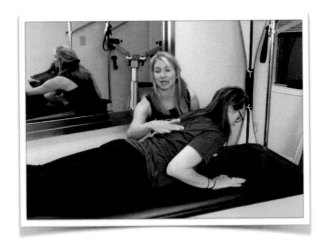

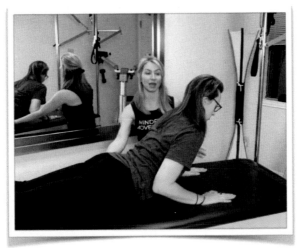

- Exhale, with control, and lower the body back down to the mat returning to your starting position.

**Need Extra Help:** Press into the forearms during extension rather than the palms.

**Precautions:** Don't forget to co-contract your deep abdominals and pelvic floor as your perform this exercise. If your shoulder blades are elevating toward your ears, push down into your elbows as you extend into a prone on elbows position. Try a few of these, and then re-visit the original swan and pay attention to your shoulder blades.

# Spine Stretch Side

**Starting Position:** Sit tall on top of the sits bones, legs straight and open shoulder width apart. Reach the arms out to your sides level with your shoulders and palms down.

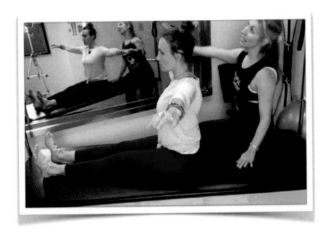

**Movement Sequence:**

- Inhale, co-contract, and reach the arms out while side-bending the body and placing one hand on the floor. The other arm will reach towards the ceiling, and the thumb will be facing towards the back of your body. Keep the body facing forward as you lean over.

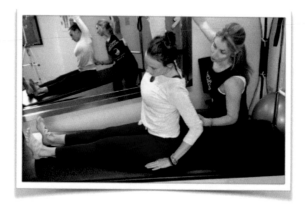

- Exhale, co-contact, and stack the spine on top of the pelvis to return to your starting position.
- Inhale, and repeat the first movement on the other side of the body.

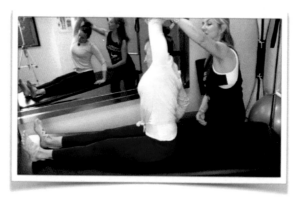

- Exhale, co-contact, and stack the spine on top of the pelvis to return to your starting position.

**Need Extra Help:** If you are unable to sit on top of your sits bones roll your mat up and sit on top of it. You may also slightly bend your knees.

**Precautions:** If you feel your lower ribs making contact with your pelvis, stop and do not push further. Start over and create length in your spine as you perform this exercise. Pay attention to see if you can go further without the contact.

# Spine Twist

**Starting Position:** Sit tall on the sits bones, legs straight and glued together. Reach the arms out to your sides level with your shoulders and palms down.

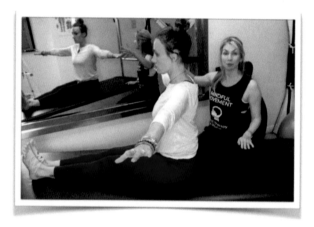

**Movement Sequence:**

- Inhale, co-contract, and root the sits bones into the mat. Rotate the spine left pulsing twice with a sniffing breath.

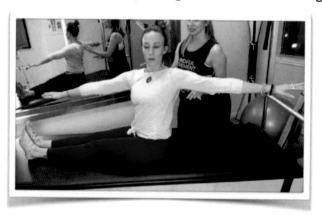

Retrain The Brain—The Dunn Method

- Exhale, return to the starting position with the weight centered on the sits bones.
- Inhale, and rotate the spine to the right, pulsing the spine twice with a sniffing breath.

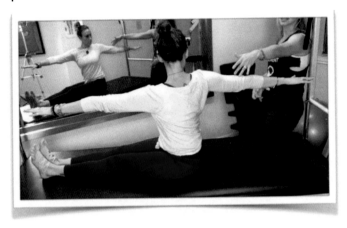

- Exhale, return to the starting position with the weight centered on the sits bones.

**Need Extra Help:** If you are unable to sit on top of your sits bones, roll your mat up and sit on top of it. You may also slightly bend your knees.

**Precautions:** It is important to create stability in the core with the co-contraction in this exercise. Maintain length in your spine in the mid range neutral position as you twist.

# Side Leg Lifts

**Starting Position:** Lie on your side with the torso and head along the back edge of the mat. Flex the hips to bring the feet in line with the front of the mat. Place your head on your lower arm as a pillow. Reach the top foot out so that it lines up with the bottom foot. This will create a small opening under the waistline that is touching the mat.

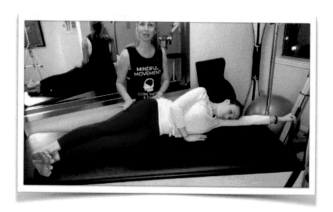

**Movement Sequence:**

- Inhale, and lift the top leg up towards the ceiling creasing at the top of the thigh. Reach the leg only as high as you can while keeping the waistline long and the hip bones and shoulders stacked.

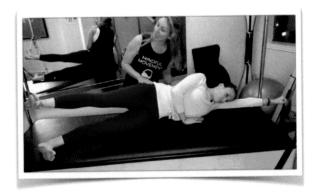

- Exhale, and lower the leg back to the starting position.
- Turn over and perform the same exercise with the other leg.

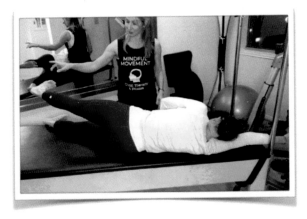

**Need Extra Help:** Try bending the bottom leg for extra support.

**Precautions:** Keep your pelvis stable and do not pivot forward or backwards. You can start this exercise with your back against the wall.

# Swimming

**Starting Position:** Lie on your stomach with arms reaching overhead and legs straight.

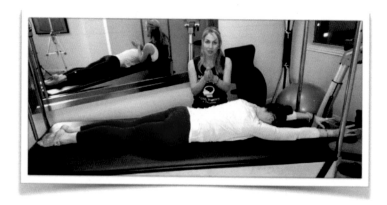

**Movement Sequence:**

- Inhale to prepare mentally.
- Exhale, co-contract, and float both arms and legs slightly off the floor. Look towards the floor and draw your scapulae down your back. Begin with one arm and the opposite leg higher than the other arm and leg.

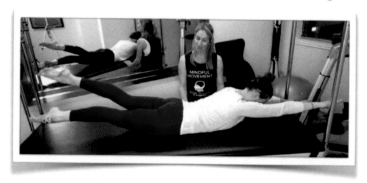

- Switch the arms and legs quickly without losing balance on the center of the torso. Inhale for two strokes and exhale for two strokes.

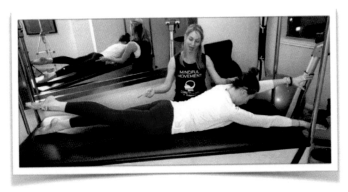

**Need Extra Help:** Just move the arms or just move the legs.

**Precautions:** Engage your deep abdominals and pull your belly button away from the floor to avoid arching your lower back

This concludes the exercises in this book.

To access the videos of each exercise, follow the link:

https://pilatestothrive.com/backpain/

Turn the page for our bonus chapter with lots of tips and resources to help you on your journey to retrain your brain to solve back pain.

# Bonus Chapter

First, I want to thank my mentors in the Physical Therapy, Pilates and fitness industries that I have studied directly with over the years. The following is a list of manual therapists that shaped my hands on skills. I do not have their proper credentials, but wish to recognize them for the training and guidance they provided. They are listed in chronological order:

- Bob Rowe, PT (in PT school)
- Brian Mulligan, PT
- Chris Kime, PT
- Chris Greetham, PT
- Chris Showalter, PT
- Bob Sprague, PT
- Chad Cook, PT
- Bob Flemming, PT
- Alan Weismantle, PT
- John Barnes, PT
- Gavin Hamer, PT
- Tom Myers

The Pilates Industry showed me a different way of teaching exercise to my clients. I am forever grateful for that one "hang up" phone call from Dr Thom that questioned my Pilates experience... Thanks also to the following:

- Thomas Werner, PT, PhD
- Barbara Wintroub
- Madeline Black
- Sherry Betz, PT
- Brent Anderson, PT
- Elizabeth Larkim

The Gyrotonic Expansion System has offered a unique learning experience for both my mind and my body. Thanks to the following for bringing such wisdom to the fitness industry:

- Donna Place
- Uwe Herbstreit, PT
- Paul Horvath, PT
- Juergen Bamberger
- Amy El

Thanks to our models:

- Dr. Jared Aguilar, PT, DPT
- Megan Strawn

I know there are many I am leaving out from the past 20+ years! Thank y'all!

# Retrain The Brain—The Dunn Method

Low Back Pain is the #1 reason why one misses work.

- 80% of Americans will experience an episode of back pain.
- 65% of them will have a re-occurrence of back pain in 1 year.
- 40% will have a re-occurrence of back pain in 4 years.
- 10-15% will become chronically disabled.

A few quick tips to consider:

- Avoid wearing high heels.
- Wear sensible footwear.
- Avoid sleeping on your stomach.
- Stay hydrated.
- Sit with both feet flat on the floor (slightly in front of the knees).
- Do not sit on the toilet any longer than you have to (Leave the cell phones in the other room).
- Do not ignore your low back pain.
- Proper exercise is important.

Do not skip the basics outlined in this book. If you exercise your big muscles instead of the deep core muscles, you can easily strain your back. However, the endorphins are released and it might feel good at the time. A flare up is thus often reported a day or 2 later.

# Retrain The Brain—The Dunn Method

I have been sharing information on my blog for a few years and want to provide the links to a few of our most popular. These blogs offer tips for sleeping positions, sitting in the bleachers, how to use a pool noodle in the car while driving, etc.:

- https://therapyandpilates.com/mattress-wars-what-mattress-should-i-buy-for-back-pain/
- https://therapyandpilates.com/with-back-pain-should-i-sleep-on-my-sides-tomach-or-back/
- https://therapyandpilates.com/a-few-simple-tips-to-ease-back-pain-while-sitting-in-the-bleachers/
- https://therapyandpilates.com/unique-tip-with-a-pool-noodle-to-open-your-chest-improve-your-spinal-posture-while-driving/
- https://therapyandpilates.com/7-simple-stretches-to-release-lower-back-and-hip-pain/
- https://therapyandpilates.com/how-do-i-get-out-of-bed-with-back-pain-log-roll-technique-for-back-pain/
- https://therapyandpilates.com/the-psoas-and-the-sway-back-core-anatomy-lesson/
- https://therapyandpilates.com/i-cant-stand-up-straight-because-of-lower-back-pain-quad-stretches-in-bed/
- https://therapyandpilates.com/back-pain-6-different-ways-to-fix-your-low-back-pain-without-surgery-or-taking-pills/

Retrain The Brain—The Dunn Method

- https://therapyandpilates.com/ease-back-pain-with-these-simple-tips-without-taking-pain-pills/

  These are just a few of the blogs available at:

- https:// therapyandpilates.com/blog/

# CONNECT WITH US!!

Join our Facebook group to connect with Stephen and Cheryl, and get access to new content regularly released in the group!

https://www.facebook.com/groups/1333041483531404

If this book or video library was of value to you, please leave a review. We personally read each one, and would love to hear from you. Please visit the following link at...

https://www.amazon.com/dp/1793494614/ref=rdr_ext_tmb

Made in the USA
Columbia, SC
19 February 2021